Lecture Notes

Clinical Anaesthesia

Carl L. Gwinnutt
MB BS MRCS LRCP FRCA
Consultant Anaesthetist
Salford Royal Hospital NHS Foundation Trust

Honorary Clinical Lecturer in Anaesthesia
University of Manchester

Third Edition

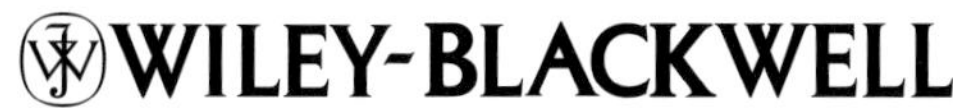

A John Wiley & Sons Ltd. Publication

Blackwell Publishing was acquired by John Wiley & Sons in February 2007. Blackwell's publishing program has been merged with Wiley's global Scientific, Technical and Medical business to form Wiley-Blackwell.

Registered office: John Wiley & Sons Ltd, The Atrium, Southern Gate, Chichester, West Sussex, PO19 8SQ, UK

Editorial offices: 9600 Garsington Road, Oxford, OX4 2DQ, UK
The Atrium, Southern Gate, Chichester, West Sussex, PO19 8SQ, UK
111 River Street, Hoboken, NJ 07030-5774, USA

For details of our global editorial offices, for customer services and for information about how to apply for permission to reuse the copyright material in this book please see our website at www.wiley.com/wiley-blackwell

Library of Congress Cataloging-in-Publication Data

Gwinnutt, Carl L.
Lecture notes. Clinical anaesthesia / Carl L. Gwinnutt. – 3rd ed.
p. ; cm.
Includes bibliographical references and index.
ISBN 978-1-4051-7038-3 (alk. paper)
1. Anesthesiology. 2. Anesthesia. I. Title. II. Title: Clinical anaesthesia.
[DNLM: 1. Anesthesia. 2. Anesthetics–administration & dosage. WO 200 G9945L 2008]
RD81.G843 2008
617.9′6–dc22

2008009438

ISBN: 978-1-4051-7038-3

A catalogue record for this book is available from the British Library.

Set in 8/12 pt Stone Serif by SNP Best-set Typesetter Ltd., Hong Kong
Printed in Singapore by Fabulous Printers Pte Ltd

1 2008

Contents

Contributors

Anthony McCluskey
Consultant in Anaesthesia and Critical Care
Stockport NHS Foundation Trust
Stepping Hill Hospital
Stockport

Richard Morgan
Consultant Anaesthetist
Salford Royal Hospital NHS Foundation Trust
Salford

Professor Gary Smith
Consultant in Critical Care Medicine
Portsmouth Hospitals NHS Trust
Queen Alexandra Hospital Portsmouth

Jasmeet Soar
Consultant in Anaesthesia and Intensive Care Medicine
Southmead Hospital
North Bristol NHS Trust
Bristol

Matthew Gwinnutt
Final year medical student
University of Birmingham

Preface

When I wrote the first edition of this book, I never envisaged that 12 years later I would be writing a third edition. During this time, the role of the anaesthetist has evolved and continues to do so. Anaesthetists now have contact with the majority of patients admitted to hospital, not only providing the conditions under which surgery can be performed safely, but also playing a major role in preoperative assessment, postoperative care, acute and chronic pain management, recognition and management of the critically ill, and resuscitation.

With each edition, I have tried to reflect the changes that are happening within anaesthesia and medicine, particularly for students. The management of chronic pain has now become a well-recognized specialty in its own right and I no longer felt that justice could be done to such an increasingly important area in a book of this size. Consequently it does not feature in this edition and readers will find many other excellent texts available. In response to the invaluable feedback I have received from students and colleagues from a variety of backgrounds, I decided to change the way in which the information on anaesthesia is presented. I have done this by dividing anaesthesia into two separate chapters; the first covers the principles behind the drugs and equipment commonly used by anaesthetists while the second chapter covers the 'hands-on' aspect of the specialty. My aim was to give a simplified view of the practicalities of giving an anaesthetic, while providing an introduction to the science behind anaesthesia for those who want more details.

Trainees from many specialties now work as part of the 'Hospital at Night' team, and part of this role is to respond to requests for help with acutely ill patients that they may not be familiar with. To help with this problem, I have included a chapter on how to deal safely and effectively with this challenging group of patients, using well-established principles. Finally the chapter on the principles of critical care has been thoroughly revised and updated.

I hope you enjoy this book, but even more I hope it helps you care for your patients. If it has, tell your friends; if it hasn't tell me why and I'll try to ensure that the next edition is better still!

Acknowledgements

I would like to thank Intersurgical for Figures 2.2 and 2.4, Aircraft Medical for Figure 2.6(b), and Deltex Medical for Figure 6.4. Figures 5.3, 5.5(a,b) and 5.7(a) are reproduced with kind permission from Michael Scott and the Resuscitation Council (UK). Figure 3.16 is reproduced with kind permission of Dr. P. Ross.

I am indebted to my son Matthew Gwinnutt for his invaluable contribution. He has tirelessly reviewed the manuscript, pointing out the differences between what I felt medical students should know and what they really need to know, and then putting this into words that they will understand. Most importantly, thank you for not being afraid to point out my occasional errors.

List of abbreviations

AAGBI Association of Anaesthetists of Great Britain and Ireland
ADH antidiuretic hormone
AED automated external defibrillator
ALS advanced life support
ARDS acute respiratory distress syndrome
ASA American Society of Anesthesiologists
AT anaerobic threshold
ATN acute tubular necrosis
BNF British National Formulary
CAVH continuous arteriovenous haemofiltration
CCU coronary care unit
CNS central nervous system
COPD chronic obstructive pulmonary disease
COX cyclo-oxygenase
CPAP continuous positive airway pressure
CPR cardiopulmonary resuscitation
CPX cardiopulmonary exercise
CRT capillary refill time
CSF cerebrospinal fluid
CT computed tomography
CTZ chemoreceptor trigger zone
CVC central venous catheter
CVP central venous pressure
CVVH continuous venovenous haemofiltration
DBP diastolic blood pressure
DNaR do not attempt resuscitation
DVT deep vein thrombosis
ECF extracellular fluid
ECG electrocardiograph
ENT ear, nose, and throat
ETT exercise tolerance test
FEV_1 forced expiratory volume in 1 second
FFP fresh frozen plasma
FRC functional residual capacity
FVC forced vital capacity
GCS Glasgow Coma Scale
GFR glomerular filtration rate
GTN glyceryl trinitrate
HAFOE high airflow oxygen enrichment
HDU high dependency unit
HIV human immunodeficiency virus
HRT hormone replacement therapy
5-HT 5-hydroxytryptamine
HTLV human T-cell lymphotrophic virus
ICF intracellular fluid
ICP intracranial pressure
ICU intensive care unit
I : E ratio inspiratory : expiratory ratio
ILM intubating LMA
IM intramuscular
INR international normalized ratio
IPPV intermittent positive pressure ventilation
IR immediate release
IV intravenous
IVRA intravenous regional anaesthesia
JVP jugular venous pressure
LED light-emitting diode
LMA laryngeal mask airway
LSD lysergic acid diethylamide
MAC minimum alveolar concentration
MAP mean arterial pressure
MET metabolic equivalent
MEWSS Modified Early Warning Scoring System
MH malignant hyperpyrexia
MI myocardial infarction
MOFS multiple organ failure syndrome
MR modified release
MRI magnetic resonance imaging
MRSA methicillin-resistant *Staphylococcus aureus*
NCEPOD National Confidential Enquiry into Patient Outcome and Death
NICE National Institute for Health and Clinical Excellence
NIPPV non-invasive positive pressure ventilation
NSAID non-steroidal anti-inflammatory drug
OCP oral contraceptive pill
ODM oesophageal Doppler monitor
OTC over the counter
$PaCO_2$ arterial partial pressure of carbon dioxide

PAFC pulmonary artery flotation catheter
PaO_2 arterial partial pressure of oxygen
PCA patient-controlled anaesthesia
PCV pressure-controlled ventilation
PE pulmonary embolism
PEA pulseless electrical activity
PEEP positive end expiratory pressure
PEFR peak expiratory flow rate
PMGV piped medical gas and vacuum system
PONV postoperative nausea and vomiting
PSV pressure support ventilation
PT prothrombin time
RSI rapid-sequence induction
SBP systolic blood pressure
SIMV synchronized intermittent mandatory ventilation
SIRS systemic inflammatory response syndrome
Spo_2 peripheral oxygenation saturation
TCI target-controlled infusion
TEB thoracic electrical bioimpedance
TIVA total intravenous anaesthesia
TOF train-of-four
TPN total parenteral nutrition
VAP ventilator-associated pneumonia
VF ventricular fibrillation
VIE vacuum-insulated evaporator
V/Q ventilation/perfusion ratio
VT ventricular tachycardia

Chapter 1

Anaesthetic assessment and preparation for surgery

The nature of anaesthetists' training and experience makes them uniquely qualified to assess the inherent risks of giving an anaesthetic. Ideally, every patient should be seen by an anaesthetist prior to surgery in order to identify, manage, and minimize these risks. Traditionally, this occurred when the patient was admitted, usually the day before an elective surgical procedure. However, if at this time the patient was found to have any significant co-morbidity, surgery was often postponed, and with no time to admit a different patient operating time was wasted. Recently, in an attempt to improve efficiency, there has been a move towards admitting a patient on the day of their planned surgical procedure. This makes the situation even more difficult by further reducing the opportunity for an adequate anaesthetic assessment. This has led to significant changes in the preoperative management of patients undergoing elective surgery, including the introduction of clinics specifically for anaesthetic assessment. A variety of models of 'preoperative' or 'anaesthetic assessment' clinic exist; the following is intended to outline their principle functions. Those who require greater detail are advised to consult the document produced by the Association of Anaesthetists of Great Britain and Ireland (AAGBI) (see Useful websites).

The preoperative assessment clinic

Stage 1

Although not all patients need to be seen by an anaesthetist in a preoperative assessment clinic, all patients do need to be assessed by an appropriately trained individual. This role is frequently undertaken by nurses, who may take a history, examine the patient, and order investigations (see below) according to the local protocol. The primary aim is to identify patients who:

- have no coexisting medical problems;
- have a coexisting medical problem that is well controlled, and does not impair daily activities, for example hypertension;
- do not require any, or require only baseline, investigations (see Table 1.1);
- have no history of, or predicted anaesthetic difficulties;
- require surgery for which complications are minimal.

Having fulfilled these criteria, patients can then be listed for surgery. At this stage, the patient will usually be given preliminary information about anaesthesia, often in the form of an explanatory leaflet.

Table 1.1 Baseline investigations in patients with no evidence of concurrent disease (ASA 1).

Age of patient	Minor surgery	Intermediate surgery	Major surgery	Major 'plus' surgery
16–39	Nil	Nil	FBC	FBC, RFT
Consider	Nil	Nil	RFT, BS	Clotting, BS
40–59	Nil	Nil	FBC	FBC, RFT
Consider	ECG	ECG, FBC, BS	ECG, BS, RFT	ECG, BS, clotting
60–79	Nil	FBC	FBC, ECG, RFT	FBC, RFT, ECG
Consider	ECG	ECG, BS, RFT	BS, CXR	BS, clotting, CXR
≥80	ECG	FBC, ECG	FBC, ECG, RFT	FBC, RFT, ECG
Consider	FBC, RFT	RFT, BS	BS, CXR, clotting	BS, clotting, CXR

FBC: full blood count; RFT: renal function tests, to include sodium, potassium, urea, and creatinine; ECG: electrocardiogram; BS: random blood glucose; CXR: chest X-ray. Clotting to include prothrombin time (PT), activated partial thromboplastin time (APTT), international normalized ratio (INR). Courtesy of National Institute for Health and Clinical Excellence.

On admission, these patients will need to be seen by a member of the surgical team, to ensure that there have not been any significant changes since attending the clinic, and by the anaesthetist who will:

- confirm the findings from the preoperative assessment;
- check the results of any baseline investigations;
- explain the options for anaesthesia appropriate for the procedure;
- have the ultimate responsibility for deciding it is safe to proceed;
- obtain consent for anaesthesia.

Stage 2

Clearly not all patients are as described above. Common reasons for patients not meeting the above criteria include:

- coexisting medical problems that are previously undiagnosed, for example diabetes, hypertension;
- medical conditions that are less than optimally managed, for example angina;
- abnormal baseline investigations.

These patients will need to be sent for further investigations, for example electrocardiography (ECG), pulmonary function tests and echocardiography, or be referred to the appropriate specialist for advice or further management before being reassessed. The findings of the further investigations then dictate whether or not the patient needs to be seen by an anaesthetist.

Stage 3

Patients that will need to be seen by an anaesthetist in the preoperative clinic are those who:

- have concurrent disease, and are symptomatic despite optimal treatment;
- are known to have had previous anaesthetic difficulties, for example difficult intubation;
- are predicted to have the potential for difficulties, for example obesity;
- have a previous or family history of prolonged apnoea after anaesthesia;
- are to undergo complex surgery with or without planned admission to the intensive care unit (ICU) postoperatively.

The consultation will allow the anaesthetist to:

- make a full assessment of the patient's medical condition;
- evaluate the results of any investigations or advice from other specialists;
- request any additional investigations;
- review any previous anaesthetics given;
- decide on the most appropriate technique, for example general or regional anaesthesia;
- begin the consent process, explaining and documenting:
  - the anaesthetic options available and the potential side-effects;

  ○ the risks associated with anaesthesia;
- discuss plans for postoperative care.

As before these patients will be seen by their anaesthetist on admission who will confirm that there have not been any significant changes since being seen in the clinic, answer any further questions that the patient may have about anaesthesia, and obtain informed consent.

The ultimate aim is to ensure that once a patient is admitted for surgery, their intended procedure is not cancelled as a result of them being deemed 'unfit' or because their medical condition has not been adequately investigated. Clearly the time between the patient being seen in the assessment clinic and the date of admission for surgery cannot be excessive; 4–6 weeks is usually acceptable.

The anaesthetic assessment

The anaesthetic assessment consists of taking a history from, and examining, each patient, followed by any appropriate investigations. When performed by non-anaesthetic staff, a protocol is often used to ensure all the relevant areas are covered. This section concentrates on features of particular relevance to the anaesthetist.

Present and past medical history

Within the patient's medical history aspects relating to the cardiovascular and respiratory systems are relatively more important to the anaesthetist than the other areas.

Cardiovascular system

Enquire specifically about symptoms of:
- ischaemic heart disease;
- heart failure;
- hypertension;
- valvular heart disease;
- conduction defects, arrhythmias;
- peripheral vascular disease, previous deep venous thrombosis (DVT) or pulmonary embolus (PE).

Patients with a proven history of myocardial infarction (MI) are at a greater risk of further infarction perioperatively. The risk of re-infarction falls as the time elapsed since the original event increases. The point at which the risk has fallen to an acceptable level, or to that of a patient with no previous history of MI, varies between individual patients. For a patient with an uncomplicated MI and a normal exercise tolerance test (ETT), elective surgery may only need to be delayed by 6–8 weeks. The American Heart Association has produced guidance for perioperative cardiovascular evaluation (see Useful websites).

Heart failure is one of the most important predictors of perioperative complications, mainly as an increased risk of perioperative cardiac morbidity and mortality. Its severity is best described using a recognized scale, for example the New York Heart Association classification (NYHA) (Table 1.2).

Untreated or poorly controlled hypertension may lead to exaggerated cardiovascular responses during anaesthesia. Both hypertension and hypotension can be precipitated, which increase the risk of myocardial and cerebral ischaemia. The severity of hypertension will determine the action required:

- *Mild (SBP 140–159 mmHg, DBP 90–99 mmHg)* No evidence that delaying surgery for treatment affects outcome.
- *Moderate (SBP 160–179 mmHg, DBP 100–109 mmHg)* Consider review of treatment. If unchanged, requires close monitoring to avoid swings during anaesthesia and surgery.
- *Severe (SBP >180 mmHg, DBP >109 mmHg)* With a BP this high, elective surgery should be postponed due to the significant risk of myocardial ischaemia, arrhythmias, and intracerebral haemorrhage. In an emergency, it will require acute control in conjunction with invasive monitoring.

Respiratory system

Enquire specifically about symptoms of:
- chronic obstructive pulmonary disease (COPD):
- chronic bronchitis;
- emphysema;
- asthma;

Table 1.2 New York Heart Association classification of cardiac function compared with the Specific Activity Scale.

NYHA functional classification		Specific Activity Scale classification
Class I	Cardiac disease without limitation of physical activity No fatigue, palpitations, dyspnoea or angina	Can perform activities requiring ≥7 METs Jog/walk at 5 mph, ski, play squash or basketball, shovel soil
Class II	Cardiac disease resulting in slight limitation of physical activity Asymptomatic at rest, ordinary physical activity causes fatigue, palpitations, dyspnoea, or angina	Can perform activities requiring ≥5 but <7 METs Walk at 4 mph on level ground, garden, rake, weed, have sexual intercourse without stopping
Class III	Cardiac disease causing marked limitation of physical activity Asymptomatic at rest, less than ordinary activity causes fatigue, palpitations, dyspnoea, or angina	Can perform activities requiring ≥2 but <5 METs Perform most household chores, play golf, push the lawnmower, shower
Class IV	Cardiac disease limiting any physical activity Symptoms of heart failure or angina at rest, increased with any physical activity	Patients cannot perform activities requiring ≥2 METs Cannot dress without stopping because of symptoms; cannot perform any class III activities

- infection;
- restrictive lung disease.

Patients with pre-existing lung disease are at increased risk of postoperative chest infections, particularly if they are also obese, or undergoing upper abdominal or thoracic surgery. If an acute upper respiratory tract infection is present, anaesthesia and surgery should be postponed unless it is for a life-threatening condition.

Assessment of exercise tolerance

Exercise capacity has long been recognized as a good predictor of postoperative morbidity and mortality. This is because similar physiological responses can be observed during exercise and after surgery, namely an increase in cardiac output and oxygen delivery to meet the increase in tissue oxygen demand. An indication of cardiac and respiratory reserves can be obtained by asking the patient about their ability to perform everyday physical activities before having to stop because of symptoms of chest pain, shortness of breath, etc. For example:

- How far can you walk on the flat?
- How far can you walk uphill?
- How many stairs can you climb before stopping?
- Could you run for a bus?
- Are you able to do the shopping?
- Are you able to do housework?
- Are you able to care for yourself?

The problem with such questions is that they are very subjective, dependent on the patient's motivation, and patients often tend to overestimate their abilities!

The assessment can be made more objective by reference to The Specific Activity Scale (Table 1.2). Common physical activities are graded in terms of their metabolic equivalents of activity or 'METs', with 1 MET being the energy (or more accurately oxygen) used at rest. The more strenuous the activity, the greater number of METs. This is not specific for each patient but serves as a useful guide, and once again relies on the patient's assessment of their activity.

Cardiopulmonary exercise testing

Cardiopulmonary exercise (CPX) testing objectively determines each patient's ability to increase oxygen delivery under controlled conditions and thereby makes a preoperative assessment of their fitness. Consequently, high-risk patients can be identified, allowing appropriate preparation to be made for their perioperative management.

To perform a CPX test, patients exercise using a bicycle ergometer, against an increasing resistance (like peddling uphill), whilst breathing through a mouthpiece. The volume and composition of inhaled and exhaled gases are monitored and analysed to determine oxygen uptake, carbon dioxide production, respiratory rate, tidal volume, and minute ventilation. The patient's oxygen saturation and ECG are also usually monitored. The principle of the test is that during exercise, oxygen consumption (VO_2, mL/min/kg) is the same as carbon dioxide production (VCO_2). As the intensity of exercise increases, a point is reached where oxygen delivery can no longer meet metabolic demand, and anaerobic metabolism starts. At this point, CO_2 production exceeds oxygen consumption; this is termed the 'anaerobic threshold' (AT). If the intensity of exercise increases further, the oxygen consumption will eventually plateau (VO_2 max), which equates to the peak aerobic capacity. Many assessments of fitness measure the AT as it occurs before VO_2 max, is more easily achieved by the elderly, and is less influenced by patient motivation. The lower the AT, the less cardiopulmonary reserve the patient has and the greater risk of postoperative morbidity and mortality. Table 1.3 shows values that have been used to predict risk and the need for an increased level of care postoperatively.

Unfortunately, not all patients can be assessed in this way; for example, those with severe musculoskeletal dysfunction may not be able to exercise to the limit of their cardiorespiratory reserve. In such circumstances, further investigations will be required. The most readily available method of non-invasive assessment of cardiac function in patients is some type of echocardiography (see below).

Other conditions in a patient's medical history which are of importance include:

- *Indigestion, heartburn, and reflux* Possibility of a hiatus hernia. If exacerbated on bending forward or lying flat, this increases the risk of regurgitation and aspiration.
- *Rheumatoid disease* Limited movement of joints makes positioning for surgery difficult. Cervical spine and temporo-mandibular joint involvement may complicate airway management. There is often a chronic anaemia.
- *Diabetes* An increased incidence of ischaemic heart disease, renal dysfunction, and autonomic and peripheral neuropathy. Increased risk of intra- and postoperative complications, particularly hypotension and infections.
- *Neuromuscular disorders* Poor respiratory function (forced vital capacity (FVC) <1 L) predisposes to chest infection and the possibility of the need for ventilatory support postoperatively. Poor bulbar function predisposes to aspiration. Care when using muscle relaxants. Consider regional anaesthesia.
- *Chronic renal failure* Anaemia and electrolyte abnormalities. Altered drug excretion restricts the choice of anaesthetic drugs. Surgery and dialysis treatments need to be coordinated.
- *Jaundice* Altered drug metabolism, coagulopathy. Care with opioid administration.

Previous anaesthetics and operations

These have usually occurred in hospitals or, occasionally in the past, dental surgeries. Enquire about any perioperative problems, for example nausea, vomiting, dreams, awareness, jaundice. Ask if any information was given postoperatively, for example difficulty with intubation, delayed recovery. Whenever possible, check the records of previous anaesthetics to rule out or clarify problems such as difficulties with intubation, allergy to drugs given, or adverse reactions (e.g. malignant hyperpyrexia, see below). Some patients may have been issued with a 'Medic Alert'-type bracelet or similar device giving details or a contact number. Details of previous surgery may reveal potential anaesthetic problems, for example cardiac, pulmonary, or cervical spine surgery.

Table 1.3 Anaerobic threshold (AT) values used to predict risk and the need for an increased level of care postoperatively.

AT >14 ml/min/kg	No specific risk, ward-based care
AT 11–14 ml/min/kg	Low risk, requires HDU care postoperatively
AT <11 ml/min/kg	High risk, requires ITU care postoperatively
Basal oxygen consumption	3.5 ml/kg/min

Family history

All patients should be asked whether any family members have experienced problems with anaesthesia; for example, a history of prolonged apnoea suggests pseudocholinesterase deficiency (see page 39), and an unexplained death suggests malignant hyperpyrexia (MH; see page 84). Elective surgery should be postponed if any conditions are identified while the patient is investigated appropriately. In the emergency situation, anaesthesia must be adjusted accordingly, for example by avoidance of triggering drugs in a patient with a potential or actual family history of MH.

Drug history and allergies

Identify all medications, both prescribed and over the counter (OTC)), including complementary and alternative medicines. Patients will often forget to mention the oral contraceptive pill (OCP) and hormone replacement therapy (HRT) unless specifically asked. On the whole, the number of medications taken rises with age. Many commonly prescribed drugs, for example beta-blockers, have important interactions with drugs used during anaesthesia. These can be identified by consulting a current British National Formulary (BNF), or the BNF website. Allergies to drugs, topical preparations (e.g. iodine), adhesive dressings, and foodstuffs should be noted.

Social history

• *Smoking* Ascertain the amount of tobacco smoked. This is usually calculated as the number of pack years; number of packs smoked each day × number of years smoked. This gives an idea of the total amount smoked and allows comparision from one person to another. Carboxyhaemoglobin reduces oxygen carriage, and nicotine stimulates the sympathetic nervous system causing tachycardia, hypertension, and coronary artery narrowing. As well as the long-term risks of smoking, i.e. chronic lung disease and carcinoma, smokers also have a significantly increased risk of postoperative chest infections. Stopping smoking before anaesthesia reduces the risk of perioperative complications; the further in advance, the better. As a guide, stopping for 8 weeks improves the airways; for 2 weeks reduces their irritability; and for as little as 24 h before anaesthesia decreases carboxyhaemoglobin levels. Help and advice should be available at the preoperative assessment clinic.

• *Alcohol* This is measured as units consumed per week: >50 units/week causes induction of liver enzymes and tolerance to anaesthetic drugs. The risk of alcohol withdrawal syndrome postoperatively must be considered.

• *Drugs* Ask specifically about the use of drugs for recreational purposes, including type, frequency, and route of administration. This group of patients is at risk of infection with hepatitis B and human immunodeficiency virus (HIV). There can be difficulty with venous access following IV drug abuse due to widespread thrombosis of veins. Withdrawal syndromes can occur postoperatively.

• *Pregnancy* The date of the last menstrual period should be noted in all women of childbearing age. The anaesthetist may be the only person in theatre able to give this information if X-rays are required. Anaesthesia increases the risk of inducing a spontaneous abortion in early pregnancy. There is an increased risk of regurgitation and aspiration in late pregnancy. Elective surgery is best postponed until after delivery.

The examination

This concentrates on the cardiovascular and respiratory systems; the remaining systems are examined if problems relevant to anaesthesia have been identified in the history. At the end of the examination, the patient's airway is assessed to try and identify any potential problems. If a regional anaesthetic is planned, the appropriate anatomy (e.g. lumbar spine for central neural block) is examined.

Cardiovascular system

Examine specifically for signs of:

• arrhythmias;
• heart failure;

- hypertension;
- valvular heart disease;
- peripheral vascular disease.

Don't forget to inspect the peripheral veins to identify any potential problems with IV access.

Respiratory system

Examine specifically for signs of:

- respiratory failure;
- impaired ventilation;
- collapse, consolidation, pleural effusion;
- additional or absent breath sounds.

Nervous system

Chronic disease of the peripheral and central nervous systems should be identified, and any evidence of motor or sensory impairment recorded. It must be remembered that some disorders will affect the cardiovascular and respiratory systems, for example dystrophia myotonica and multiple sclerosis.

Musculoskeletal system

Note any restriction of movement and deformity if a patient has connective tissue disorders. Patients suffering from chronic rheumatoid disease frequently have a reduced muscle mass, peripheral neuropathies, and pulmonary involvement. Particular attention should be paid to the patient's cervical spine and temporo-mandibular joints (see below).

The airway

The airway of all patients must be assessed, in order to try to predict those patients who may be difficult to intubate.

Observation of the patient's anatomy

Look for:

- limitation of mouth opening;
- a receding mandible;
- position, number, and health of teeth;
- size of the tongue;
- soft tissue swelling at the front of the neck;
- deviation of the larynx or trachea;
- limitations in flexion and extension of the cervical spine.

Finding any of these suggests that intubation may be more difficult. However, it must be remembered that all of these are subjective.

Simple bedside tests

- *Mallampati criteria* The patient, sitting upright, is asked to open their mouth and maximally protrude their tongue. The view of the pharyngeal structures is noted and graded I–IV (Fig. 1.1). Grades III and IV suggest difficult intubation.
- *Thyromental distance* With the head fully extended on the neck, the distance between the bony point of the chin and the prominence of the thyroid cartilage is measured (Fig. 1.2). A distance of <7 cm suggests difficult intubation.
- *Wilson score* Increasing weight, a reduction in head and neck movement, reduced mouth opening, and the presence of a receding mandible or buck-teeth all predispose to increased difficulty with intubation.
- *Calder test* The patient is asked to protrude the mandible as far as possible. The lower incisors will lie either anterior to, aligned with, or posterior to the upper incisors. The latter two suggest a reduced view at laryngoscopy.

None of these tests, alone or in combination, will predict all difficult intubations. A Mallampati grade III or IV with a thyromental distance of <7 cm will predict 80% of difficult intubations. If problems are anticipated, anaesthesia should be planned accordingly. If intubation proves to be difficult, it must be recorded in a prominent place in the patient's notes and the patient informed.

Investigations

There is little evidence to support 'routine' investigations, and so an investigation should only be ordered if the result would affect the patient's management. *In patients with no evidence of concurrent disease* (ASA 1, see below), preoperative

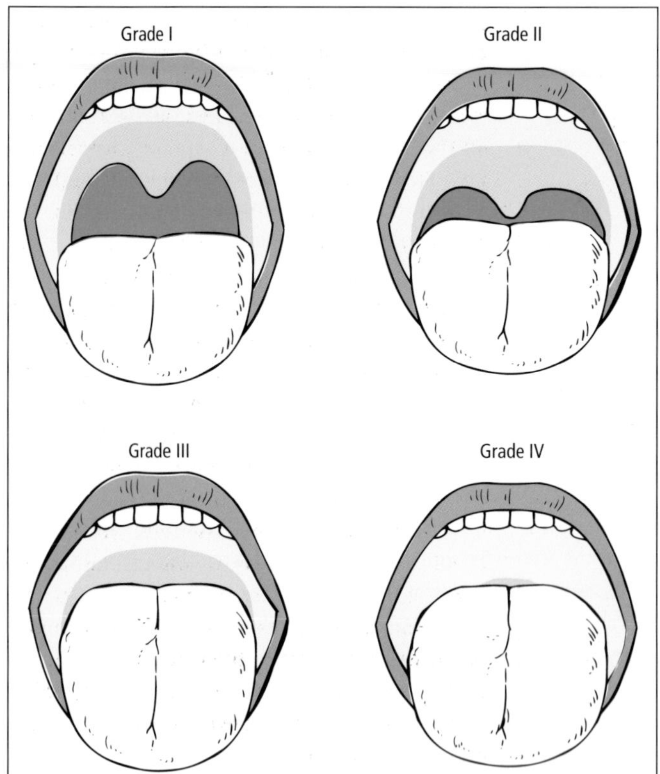

Figure 1.1 The pharyngeal structures seen during the Mallampati assessment.

investigations will depend on the extent of surgery and the age of the patient. A synopsis of the current guidelines for these patients, issued by the National Institute for Health and Clinical Excellence (NICE), is shown in Table 1.1. For each age group and grade of surgery, the upper entry shows 'tests recommended' and the lower entry 'tests to be considered' (depending on patient characteristics). Dipstick urinalysis needs only to be performed in symptomatic individuals.

Additional investigations

The following is a guide for when to request some of the common preoperative investigations. Again the need for these will depend on the grade of surgery and the age of the patient. Further information can be found in Clinical Guideline 3, published by NICE (see Useful websites).

- *Urea and electrolytes*: patients taking digoxin, diuretics, steroids, and those with diabetes, renal disease, vomiting, diarrhoea.
- *Liver function tests*: known hepatic disease, a history of a high alcohol intake (>50 units/week), metastatic disease, or evidence of malnutrition.
- *Blood sugar*: diabetics, severe peripheral arterial disease, or taking long-term steroids.
- *ECG*: hypertensive, with symptoms or signs of ischaemic heart disease, a cardiac arrhythmia, or diabetics >40 years of age.
- *Chest X-ray*: symptoms or signs of cardiac or respiratory disease, or suspected or known malignancy, where thoracic surgery is planned, or in those from areas of endemic tuberculosis who have not had a chest X-ray in the last year.
- *Pulmonary function tests*: dyspnoea on mild exertion, COPD, or asthma. Measure peak expiratory flow rate (PEFR), forced expiratory volume in 1 second (FEV_1), and FVC. Patients who are dyspnoeic

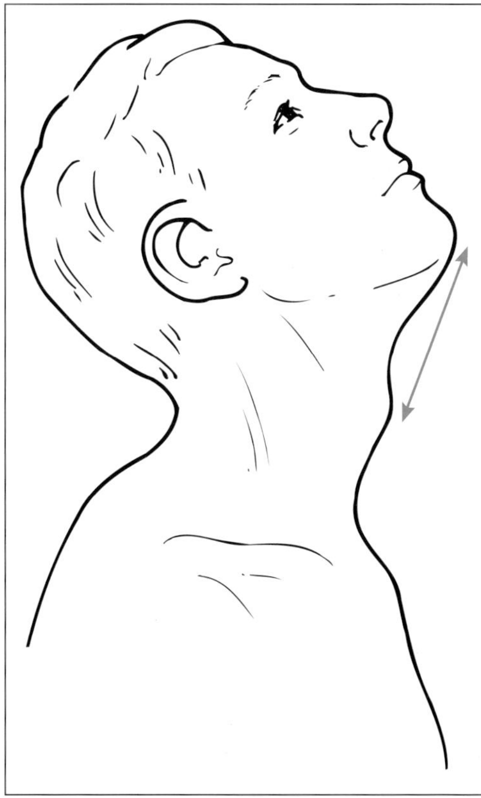

Figure 1.2 The thyromental distance.

or cyanosed at rest, found to have an FEV_1 <60% predicted, or are to have thoracic surgery, should also have arterial blood gas analysed while breathing air.

• *Coagulation screen*: anticoagulant therapy, a history of a bleeding diatheses, or a history of liver disease or jaundice.

• *Sickle-cell screen (Sickledex)*: a family history of sickle-cell disease or where ethnicity increases the risk of sickle-cell disease. If positive, electrophoresis will be required for definitive diagnosis.

• *Cervical spine X-ray*: rheumatoid arthritis, a history of major trauma or surgery to the neck, or when difficult intubation is predicted.

Echocardiography

This is becoming increasingly recognized as a useful tool to assess left ventricular function in patients with ischaemic or valvular heart disease, but whose exercise ability is limited, for example by severe osteoarthritis. The left ventricular ejection fraction can be calculated, and contractility and ventricular wall motion abnormalities identified. Similarly, ventricular function post-MI can be assessed. In patients with valvular lesions, the degree of dysfunction (regurgitation and/or stenosis) can be assessed. In aortic stenosis, the valve (aperture) area can be measured and the pressure gradient across the valve, which is a good indication of the severity of the disease, can be calculated. As an echocardiogram is performed in patients at rest, it does not give any indication of what happens when metabolic demand is increased. A stress echocardiogram can be performed to simulate exercise and hence the conditions a patient may encounter during anaesthesia or after surgery. This is often achieved by administering an inotrope, for example dobutamine, which increases the heart rate and myocardial work while any changes in myocardial performance are monitored (dobutamine stress echocardiography).

Medical referral

Patients with significant medical (or surgical) co-morbidities should be identified in the preoperative assessment clinic, not on the day of admission, to allow time for adequate investigation and management. Clearly a wide spectrum of conditions exists; the following are examples of some of the more commonly encountered that may need specialist advice.

Cardiovascular disease

• Untreated or poorly controlled hypertension or heart failure.

• Symptomatic ischaemic heart disease, despite treatment (unstable angina).

• Arrhythmias: uncontrolled atrial fibrillation, paroxysmal supraventricular tachycardia, and second and third degree heart block.

• Symptomatic or newly diagnosed valvular heart disease, or congenital heart disease.

Respiratory disease

- COPD, particularly if dyspnoeic at rest.
- Bronchiectasis.
- Asthmatics who are unstable, taking oral steroids or have an FEV_1 <60% predicted.

Endocrine disorders

- Insulin-dependent and non-insulin dependent diabetics who have ketonuria, glycated haemoglobin (HbA1c) >10%, or a random blood sugar >12 mmol/L. Local policy will dictate referral of stable diabetics for perioperative management.
- Hypo- or hyperthyroidism symptomatic on current treatment.
- Cushing's or Addison's disease.
- Hypopituitarism.

Renal disease

- Chronic renal failure.
- Patients undergoing renal replacement therapy.

Haematological disorders

- Bleeding diatheses, for example haemophilia, thrombocytopenia.
- Therapeutic anticoagulation.
- Haemoglobinopathies.
- Polycythaemia.
- Haemolytic anaemias.
- Leukaemias.

Risk associated with anaesthesia and surgery

One of the most commonly asked questions of anaesthetists is '*What are the risks of having an anaesthetic?*' These can be divided into two main groups.

Minor

These are not life threatening and can occur even when anaesthesia has apparently been uneventful. Although classed as minor, the patient may not share this view. They include:

- failed IV access;
- cut lip, damage to teeth, caps, crowns;
- sore throat;
- headache;
- postoperative nausea and vomiting (PONV);
- retention of urine.

Major

These may be life-threatening events. They include but are not limited to:

- aspiration of gastric contents;
- hypoxic brain injury;
- MI;
- cerebrovascular accident;
- nerve injury;
- chest infection;
- renal failure;
- death.

In the UK, the Confidential Enquiry into Perioperative Deaths (CEPOD 1987) revealed an *overall* perioperative mortality of 0.7% in approximately 500 000 operations. Anaesthesia was considered to have been a contributing factor in 410 deaths (0.08%), but was judged *completely* responsible in only three cases—a primary mortality rate of 1:185 000 operations. Upon analysis of the deaths where anaesthesia contributed, the predominant factor was human error.

Clearly, anaesthesia itself is very safe, particularly in those patients who are otherwise well. Apart from human error, the most likely risk is from an adverse drug reaction or drug interaction. However, anaesthesia rarely occurs in isolation and, when the risks of the surgical procedure and those due to pre-existing disease are combined, the risks of morbidity and mortality are increased. Not surprisingly, a number of methods have been described to try and quantify these risks.

Risk indicators

The most widely used scale for estimating risk is the American Society of Anesthesiologists (ASA) classification of the patient's physical status. The patient is assigned to a category from 1 to 5 depending on any physical disturbance caused by either the disease process for which surgery is being performed or any other pre-existing disease. It is relatively subjective and does not take into

Table 1.4 ASA physical status scale.

Class	Physical status	Absolute mortality (%)
I	A healthy patient with no organic or psychological disease process. The pathological process for which the operation is being performed is localized and causes no systemic upset	0.1
II	A patient with a mild to moderate systemic disease process, caused by the condition to be treated surgically or another pathological process, that does not limit the patient's activities in any way, e.g. treated hypertensive, stable diabetic. Patients aged >80 years are automatically placed in class II	0.2
III	A patient with severe systemic disease from any cause that imposes a definite functional limitation on activity, e.g. ischaemic heart disease, chronic obstructive lung disease	1.8
IV	A patient with a severe systemic disease that is a constant threat to life, e.g. unstable angina	7.8
V	A moribund patient unlikely to survive 24 h with or without surgery	9.4

Note: 'E' may be added to signify an emergency operation.

account the type of surgery being undertaken, which leads to a degree of variability between scorers. However, patients placed in higher categories are at increased overall risk of perioperative mortality (Table 1.4).

Multifactorial risk indicators

The leading cause of death after surgery is MI, and significant morbidity results from non-fatal infarction, particularly in patients with pre-existing heart disease. Attempts have been made to identify factors that will predict those at risk. One system is the Goldman Cardiac Risk Index, used in patients with pre-existing cardiac disease undergoing non-cardiac surgery. Factors in their history, examination, ECG, general status, and type of surgery are awarded points (Table 1.5).

The points total is used to assign patients to a class from I to IV according to their risk of a

Table 1.5 Goldman Cardiac Risk Index.

	Points
History	
Age >70 years	5
Myocardial infarction within 6 months	10
Examination	
Third heart sound (gallop rhythm), raised JVP	11
Significant aortic stenosis	3
ECG	
Rhythm other than sinus, or presence of premature atrial complexes	7
>5 ventricular ectopics per minute	7
General condition	
PaO_2 <8 kPa or $PaCO_2$ >7.5 kPa on air	
K^+ <3.0 mmol/L; HCO_3^- <20 mmol/L	
Urea >8.5 mmol/L; creatinine >200 mmol/L	
Chronic liver disease	
Bedridden from non-cardiac cause	
For each criterion	3
Operation	
Intraperitoneal, intrathoracic, aortic	3
Emergency surgery	4

JVP, jugular venous pressure.

perioperative cardiac event, namely MI, pulmonary oedema, significant arrhythmia, and death:

- Class I (0–5 points) 1%
- Class II (6–12 points) 5%
- Class III (13–25 points) 16%
- Class IV (⩾26 points) 56%

This has been shown to be a more accurate predictor of postoperative morbidity than the ASA classification.

As well as the risks of perioperative complications varying with the type and severity of pre-existing cardiac disease, different operations also carry their own varying levels of inherent risks, for example carpal tunnel decompression carries less risk than a hip replacement, which in turn carries less risk than aortic aneurysm surgery. This is clearly demonstrated in Table 1.6 where overall risk of cardiac complications is calculated based upon the Goldman score and grade of surgery. Basically this can be summarized as 'the sicker the patient and the bigger the operation, the greater the risk'. Major cardiac complications include MI, cardiogenic pulmonary oedema, ventricular tachycardia, or cardiac death.

Assessing patients as 'low risk' is no more of a guarantee that complications will not occur than 'high risk' means they will occur; it is only a guideline and indicator of probability. For patients who suffer a complication, the rate is 100%! Ultimately the risk/benefit ratio must be considered for each individual patient. If a patient has a certain predicted risk of complications, an operation with the potential to offer only a small benefit may be deemed not worth the risk, whereas one with the potential to offer a large benefit may in fact be undertaken. Clearly this is a decision which can only be reached after careful and thorough discussion with a patient who has been given all the relevant information.

Improving preoperative preparation by optimizing the patient's physical status, adequately resuscitating those who require emergency surgery, monitoring appropriately intraoperatively, and providing suitable postoperative care, in a high dependency unit (HDU) or ICU, has been shown to reduce patients perioperative mortality further.

Classification of operation

Traditionally, surgery was classified as being either elective or emergency. Recognizing that this was too imprecise, the National Confidential Enquiry into Perioperative Outcome and Death (NCEPOD) has identified four categories:

1 Immediate: to save life, limb, or organ. Resuscitation is simultaneous with surgery. The target time to theatre is within minutes of the decision that surgery is necessary, for example major trauma to the abdomen or thorax with uncontrolled haemorrhage, major neurovascular deficit, ruptured aortic aneurysm.

2 Urgent: acute onset or deterioration of a condition that threatens life, limb, or organ. Surgery normally takes place when resuscitation is complete. This category is subdivided into:

- Target time to theatre within 6 h of the decision to operate

Table 1.6 Overall approximate risk (%) of a major cardiac complication based on the type of surgery and the patient's cardiac risk index.

	Patient risk index score			
	Class I	Class II	Class III	Class IV
Grade of surgery	(0–5 points)	(6–12 points)	(13–25 points)	(⩾26 points)
Minor surgery	0.3	1	3	19
Major non-cardiac surgery, >40 years	1.2	4	12	48
Major non-cardiac surgery, >40 years, significant medical problem requiring consultation before surgery	3	10	30	75

- Target time to theatre within 24 h of the decision to operate.

3 Expedited: stable patient requiring early intervention. Condition not an immediate threat to life, limb, or organ. Target time to theatre is within days of the decision to operate.

4 Elective: surgery planned and booked in advance of admission to hospital. This category includes all conditions not covered in categories 1–3.

All elective and the majority of expedited cases can be assessed as previously described, but in urgent and emergency cases this will not always be possible. As much information as possible should be obtained about allergies, the patient's medical history, drugs taken regularly, and previous anaesthetics. In the trauma patient, enquire about the mechanism of injury. This may give clues to unsuspected injuries. Details may only be available from relatives and/or the ambulance crew. The cardiovascular and respiratory systems should be examined and an assessment made of any potential difficulty with intubation. Investigations should only be ordered if they would directly affect the conduct of anaesthesia. When life or limb is at stake, there will be even less or no time for assessment. All emergency patients should be assumed to have a full stomach.

Obtaining informed consent

What is consent?

Consent is an agreement by the patient to undergo a specific procedure. Even though the doctor will advise on what is required, it is only the patient who can make the decision to undergo the procedure. Although the need for consent is usually thought of as applying to surgery, it is in fact required for any breach of a patient's personal integrity, including examination, performing investigations, and administering an anaesthetic. Touching a patient without consent may lead to a claim of battery. For a patient to have capacity to give valid consent there are five prerequisites: they must have been given all the information; understand and retain it; believe it; weigh it in the balance; and then communicate their decision. The decision the patient makes does not have to appear sensible or rational to anybody else. However, every effort must be made to ensure that a highly irrational decision is not the result of a lack of, or misinterpretation of, the information given. It may of course also indicate that the patient is suffering from a mental illness. Determining capacity on these grounds is probably best placed in the hands of the courts.

Refusal of treatment by a competent adult is legally binding, even if refusal is likely to lead to the patient's death (e.g. a Jehovah's Witness refusing a blood transfusion). Although a patient can refuse treatment or choose a less than optimal option, they cannot insist on a treatment that has not been offered.

What about an unconscious patient?

This usually arises in the emergency situation, for example a patient with a severe head injury. Asking a relative or other individual to sign a consent form for surgery on the patient's behalf is not appropriate, as no one can give consent on behalf of another adult. Under these circumstances, medical staff are required to act 'in the patient's best interests'. This will mean taking into account not only the benefits of the proposed treatment, but also personal and social factors. Such information may necessitate a discussion with relatives, and the opportunity should be used to inform them of the proposed treatment and the rationale for it. The basis for any decision and how it is in the patient's best interests must be clearly documented in the patient's notes. Where treatment decisions are complex or not clear-cut, it is advisable, although not a legal requirement, to obtain and document independent medical advice.

What constitutes evidence of consent?

Most patients will be asked to sign a consent form before undergoing a procedure. However, there is no legal requirement for such before anaesthesia or surgery (or anything else). Consent may be given verbally, and this is often the case for anaesthesia; however, it is recommended that a written record of the content of the conversation be made in the patient's case notes.

What do I have to tell the patient?

Although the anaesthetist is the best judge of the type of anaesthetic for each individual, patients should be given an explanation of the choices, along with the associated risks and benefits. The amount of information will vary depending on the procedure, and should be determined by asking oneself 'what would this patient regard as relevant when coming to a decision about which, if any, of the available options to accept?' Typical information given may be:

- The environment of the anaesthetic room and who they will meet, particularly if medical students or other healthcare professionals in training will be present.
- Establishing IV access and IV infusion.
- The need for, and type of, any invasive monitoring.
- What to expect during the establishment of a regional technique.
- Being conscious throughout surgery if a regional technique alone is used, and what they may hear.
- Preoxygenation.
- Induction of anaesthesia. Although most commonly IV, occasionally it may be by inhalation.
- Where they will 'wake up'. This is usually the recovery unit, but after some surgery it may be the ICU or HDU. In these circumstances, the patient should be given the opportunity to visit the unit a few days before and meet some of the staff.
- Numbness and loss of movement after regional anaesthesia.
- The possibility of drains, catheters, and drips. Patients may misinterpret their presence as indicating unexpected problems.
- The possibility of a need for blood transfusion.
- Postoperative pain control, particularly if it requires their cooperation, for example a patient-controlled analgesia device (PCA; see pages 102–104).
- Information on any substantial risks with serious adverse consequences associated with the anaesthetic technique planned.
- Risks associated with the anaesthetic technique (see above).

Most patients will want to know the latest time that they can eat and drink before surgery, if they should take their medications as normal, and how they will manage without a drink. Some will expect or request a premed and, in these circumstances, the approximate timing, route of administration, and likely effects should be discussed. Finally, before leaving, ask if the patient has any questions or wants anything clarified further.

Having given the patient the information considered relevant to them, they must have sufficient time to think it through and come to a decision. Consequently, the process of informed consent cannot occur solely at the point of admission or, even worse, in the anaesthetic room immediately before surgery! As a result, the process usually starts in the preoperative assessment clinic when information is often given to the patient in the form of a leaflet.

Who should get consent?

From the above it is clear that the individual seeking consent must be able to provide all the necessary information for the patient and be able to answer the patient's questions. This will require the individual to be trained in, and familiar with, the procedure for which consent is sought, and is best done by a senior clinician or the person who is to perform the procedure. Complex problems may require a multidisciplinary approach to obtaining consent.

The issues around consent in children and adults who lack capacity are more complex. Further information is available in the document 'Consent for Anaesthesia' published by the AAGBI (see Useful websites section for more information).

Useful websites

http://www.aagbi.org/publications/guidelines/docs/preoperativeass01.pdf

[Preoperative assessment. The role of the anaesthetist. The Association of Anaesthetists of Great Britain and Ireland. November 2001.]

http://www.circ.ahajournals.org/cgi/content/full/116/17/1971
[ACC/AHA 2007 Guidelines on Perioperative Cardiovascular Evaluation and Care for Noncardiac Surgery: Executive Summary]

http://www.americanheart.org/downloadable/heart/1142081026765PeriopFinal.pdf
[ACC/AHA 2006 Guideline Update on Perioperative Cardiovascular Evaluation for Noncardiac Surgery: Focused Update on Perioperative Beta-Blocker Therapy. A Report of the American College of Cardiology/American Heart Association Task Force on Practice Guidelines (Writing Committee to Update the 2002 Guidelines on Perioperative Cardiovascular Evaluation for Noncardiac Surgery)]

http://www.nice.org.uk/guidance/index.jsp?action=byID&r=true&o=10920
[National Institute for Health and Clinical Excellence (NICE) guidance on preoperative tests. June 2003.]

http://info.med.yale.edu/intmed/cardio/imaging/contents.html
[Chest X-ray interpretation.]

http://www.ncepod.org.uk/
[The National Confidential Enquiry into Patient Outcome and Death (NCEPOD).]

http://www.dh.gov.uk/en/Publichealth/Scientificdevelopmentgeneticsandbioethics/Consent/index.htm
[Department of Health (UK) guidance on consent.]

http://www.bma.org.uk/ap.nsf/Content/consenttk2
[BMA consent toolkit, second edition. February 2003.]

http://www.aagbi.org/publications/guidelines/docs/consent06.pdf
[Consent for anesthesia. Revised edition 2006. The Association of Anaesthetists of Great Britain & Ireland

http://www.dca.gov.uk/menincap/legis.htm
[Mental Capacity Act 2005. Department of Constitutional Affairs.]

http://www.youranaesthetic.info/

http://www.aagbi.org/pub_patient.html#KNOW
[Patient information guides from the Association of Anaesthetists of Great Britain and Ireland and The Royal College of Anaesthetists.]

http://www.pre-op.org/index.html
[The Preoperative Association]

All websites last accessed April 2008.

Self-assessment

1.1 Describe three methods of assessing a patient's exercise capacity preoperatively.

1.2 Describe what bedside assessments you could use to try and predict difficulty with tracheal intubation.

1.3 Describe the health characteristics that define each of the five ASA grades. What ASA grade would you assign to a 67-year-old woman with type II diabetes, hypertension, a BMI of 38 and exercise tolerance of 100 m on the flat, and why?

1.4 In the preoperative assessment clinic, what investigations would you do on a 70-year-old woman, with controlled hypertension and COPD from smoking 20 cigarettes per day for 50 years, who is scheduled for a total hip replacement and why?

Chapter 2

The principles of anaesthesia

Anaesthesia is a very practical specialty, and to practise safely anaesthetists must be familiar with the equipment used. This ranges from the simple to the technical, the complexity of which is increasing relentlessly. The following is an overview of the equipment and drugs currently in use. No excuse is made for including very simple devices; even these, if used correctly, are very valuable, but if used wrongly may endanger the patient's safety.

Airway equipment

A wide variety of equipment and skills are required to ensure that the patient has a patent airway at all times. The following is a description of the equipment; a description of the skills needed to use it safely and successfully is given in Chapter 3.

Simple adjuncts

The oropharyngeal (Guedel) airway and, to a lesser extent, the nasopharyngeal airway are often used to help maintain the airway immediately after the induction of anaesthesia. However, their use does not guarantee a patent airway.

Oropharyngeal airway

These are curved plastic tubes, flattened in cross-section and flanged at the oral end (Fig. 2.1). They lie over the tongue, and prevent it from falling back into the pharynx. They are manufactured in a variety of sizes suitable for all patients, from neonates to large adults. The most common sizes are 2–4, for small to large adults, respectively. The size required is estimated by comparing the airway length with the vertical distance between the patient's incisor teeth and the angle of the jaw.

Nasopharyngeal airway

These are round, malleable plastic tubes, bevelled at the pharyngeal end and flanged at the nasal end (Fig. 2.1). They lie along the floor of the nose and curve round into the pharynx. They are sized according to their internal diameter in millimetres, and their length increases with the diameter. They are not commonly used in children, and tubes 6–8 mm in diameter are suitable for small to large adults, respectively. The correct size is estimated by comparing the airway diameter with that of the external nares.

Facemasks

These are designed to fit closely the contours of the face, and a gas-tight fit is achieved by an air-filled cuff around the edge. They are either reusable, for example the BOC anatomical facemask, and require disinfection between each patient, or are single use. Disposable masks are usually transparent,

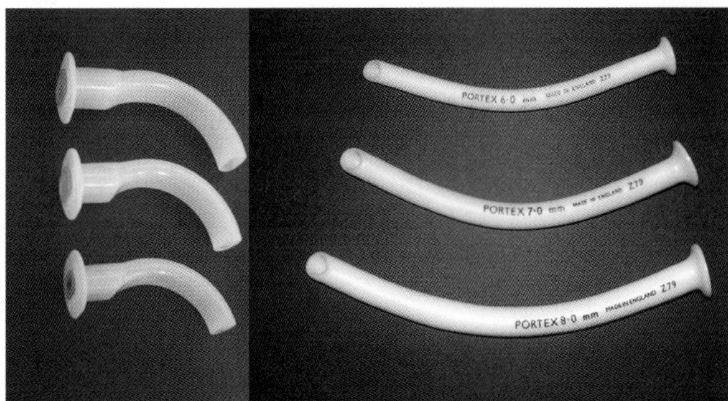

Figure 2.1 Oropharyngeal and nasopharyngeal airways.

allowing visualization of vomit, making them popular for use during resuscitation.

The laryngeal mask airway (LMA)

As its name suggests, this device consists of a 'mask' that sits over the laryngeal opening attached to a tube that protrudes from the mouth and connects directly to the anaesthetic breathing system. Around the perimeter of the mask is an inflatable cuff that helps to stabilize it and creates a seal around the laryngeal inlet. The LMA is suitable for use in all patients, from neonates to adults, as it is produced in a variety of sizes. The most commonly used in female and male adults are sizes 3, 4, and 5. It was originally designed for use in spontaneously breathing patients, but it is possible to ventilate patients via the LMA. When doing this, care must be taken to avoid high inflation pressures, otherwise leakage occurs past the cuff reducing ventilation and potentially causing gastric inflation. The original LMA (or classic LMA) is a reusable device requiring sterilization between each patient, but recent concerns about the possible risk of prion disease transmission have resulted in increasing use of disposable versions (Fig. 2.2a). There have been a number of other developments of the LMA:

- A version with a reinforced tube to prevent kinking.
- The Proseal® LMA (Fig. 2.2b): this has an additional posterior cuff to improve the seal between

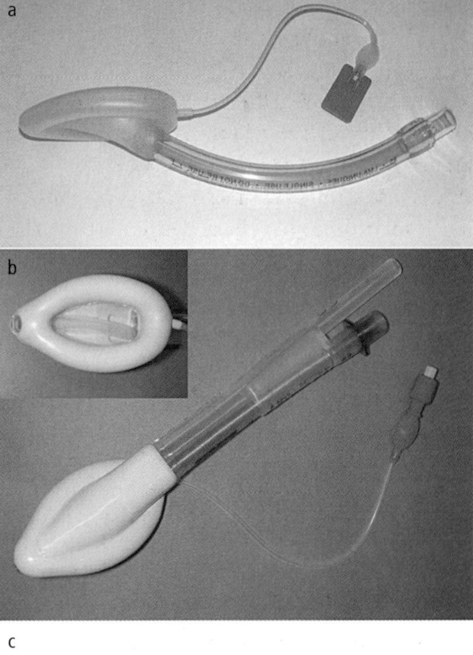

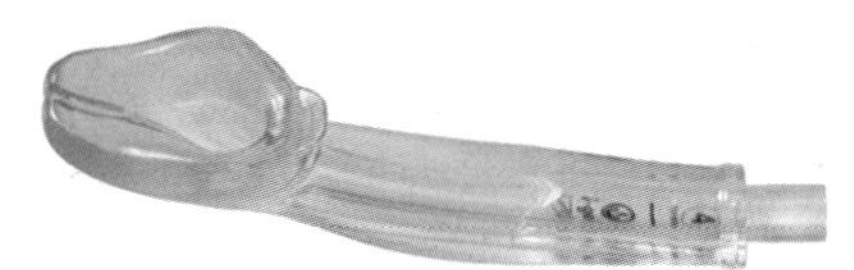

Figure 2.2 (a) Disposable laryngeal mask airway (LMA), (b) Proseal LMA, (c) i-gel supraglottic airway.

mask and larynx, and reduce leak when the patient is ventilated. It also has a secondary tube to allow drainage of gastric contents.

- The i-gel® (Fig. 2.2c): this is the latest development which uses a solid, highly malleable, gel-like material contoured to fit the perilaryngeal anatomy in place of the traditional inflatable cuff . It is single use.
- The intubating LMA (ILM; Fig. 2.3): as the name suggests, this device is used as a conduit to perform tracheal intubation without the need for laryngoscopy (see below).

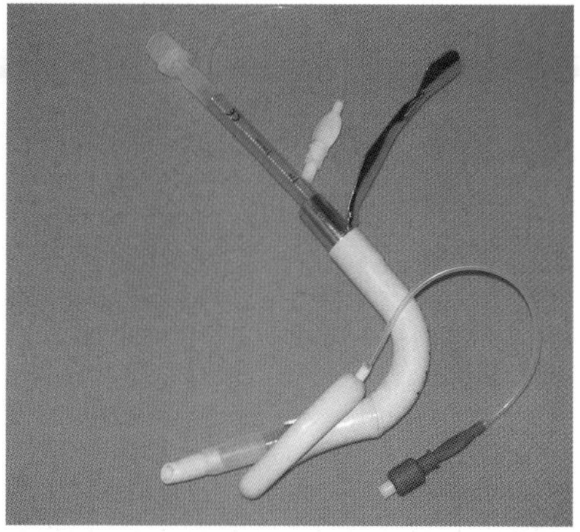

Figure 2.3 Intubating laryngeal mask airway (ILM) with a tracheal tube passing through the mask.

The ILM

This is a modification of the LMA in which the mask part is almost unchanged, but a shorter, wider metal tube with a 90° bend in it with a handle replaces the flexible tube (Fig. 2.3). It is inserted using a similar technique to that for a standard LMA, but by holding the handle rather than using one's index finger as a guide. A specially designed reinforced, cuffed, tracheal tube can then be inserted which will almost always pass into the trachea, due to the shape and position of the ILM. Once it has been confirmed that the tube lies in the trachea, the ILM can either be left in place or removed. This device has proved to be very popular in cases where direct laryngoscopy does not give a good view of the larynx and tracheal intubation fails. The most recent development is the CTrach™, in which the larynx is viewed from the mask aperture via a fibreoptic cable attached to a small monitor positioned at the proximal end of the device (Fig. 2.4).

There are also similar devices made by other companies. Increasingly, these devices are referred to as 'supraglottic airways'.

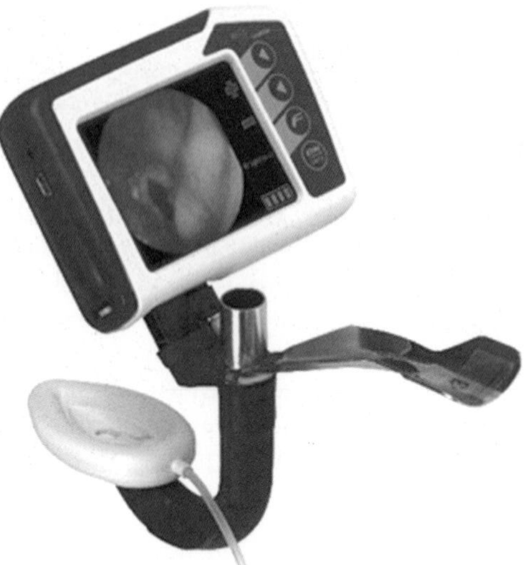

Figure 2.4 CTrach: an ILM with integrated fibreoptics to allow a view of the larynx.

Tracheal tubes

These are manufactured from plastic (PVC), and are single use to eliminate cross-infection. They are available in a range of sizes at 0.5 mm diameter intervals, making them suitable for use in all patients from neonates to adults, and long enough to be used orally or nasally. A standard 15 mm connector is provided to allow connection to the breathing system.

The tracheal tubes used during adult anaesthesia have an inflatable cuff to prevent leakage of anaesthetic gases back past the tube when positive pressure ventilation is used, and also to prevent

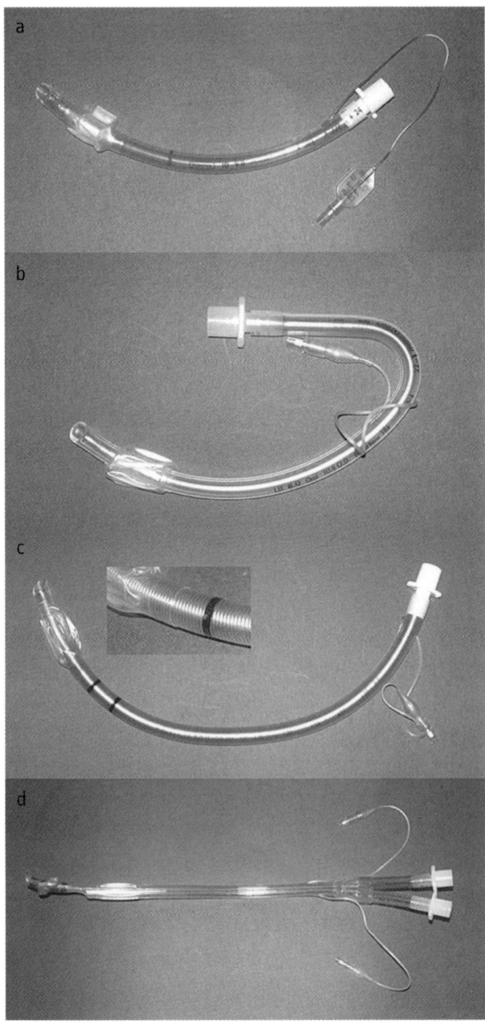

Figure 2.5 Tracheal tubes. (a) Standard PVC, (b) preformed (RAE tube), (c) reinforced tube, (d) double lumen tube

aspiration of any foreign material into the lungs. The cuff is inflated by injecting air via a pilot tube, at the distal end of which is a one-way valve to prevent deflation and a small 'balloon' to indicate when the cuff is inflated. A wide variety of specialized tubes have been developed, examples of which are shown in Fig. 2.5.

- *Preformed tubes* are used during surgery on the head and neck, and are designed to take the connections away from the surgical field.
- *Reinforced tubes* are used to prevent kinking and subsequent obstruction as a result of the positioning of the patient's head.
- *Double-lumen tubes* are effectively two tubes welded together side-by-side, with one tube extending distally beyond the other. They are used during thoracic surgery, and allow one lung to be deflated whilst ventilation is maintained via the bronchial portion in the opposite lung.
- *Uncuffed tubes* are used in children up to approximately 10 years of age as the narrowing in the subglottic region provides a natural seal.

Laryngoscopes

These are designed to allow direct visualization of the larynx to facilitate the insertion of a tracheal tube. They consist of a blade with a light at the tip, attached to a handle that contains the batteries for the light. The most popular type in use is the curved blade designed by, and named after, Sir Robert Macintosh (Fig. 2.6a). There have been many developments in the design of this device, and one of the most successful is the McCoy blade (Fig. 2.6c and d). This has a flexible tip operated by a lever adjacent to the handle which increases the elevation of the epiglottis to improve the view of the larynx. Occasionally a straight-bladed laryngoscope may be used, for example the Magill blade. The most recent development is the use of modern electronics to project the view from the tip of the blade onto a small display unit adjacent to the handle (the McGrath Scope, Fig. 2.6b) or a freestanding monitor. Such devices are intended to overcome the difficulties when the larynx cannot be seen under direct vision, making intubation difficult.

Gum elastic bougie

This is a 60 cm long malleable introducer, with a slightly angled tip. Its construction allows it to be bent into a gentle curve before it is introduced so that it can be directed blindly behind the epiglottis into the trachea. It is then rigid enough to allow a tracheal tube to be passed over it.

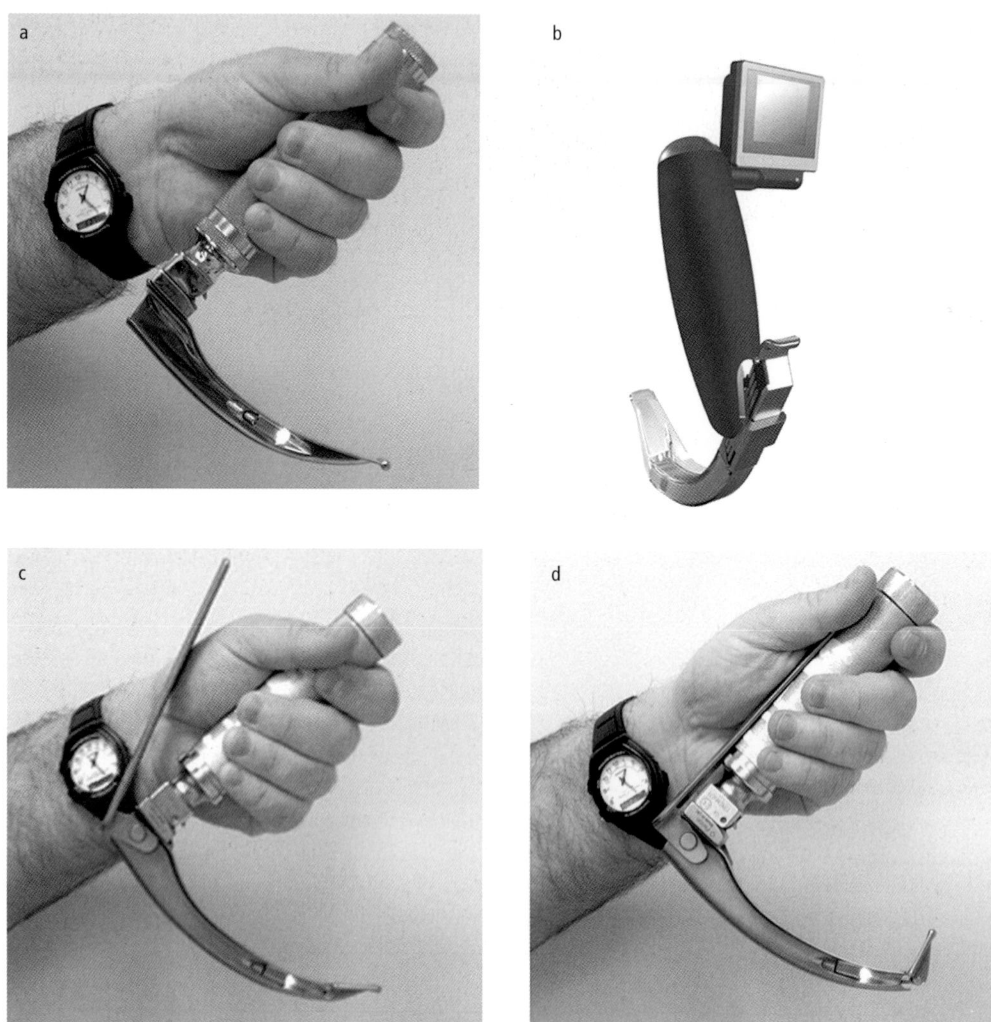

Figure 2.6 (a) Macintosh laryngoscope, (b) McGrath laryngoscope, (c and d) McCoy blade. Neutral (c) and with the tip flexed to elevate the epigottis (d).

The safe delivery of anaesthesia

The delivery of gases to the operating theatre

Most hospitals use a piped medical gas and vacuum system (PMGV) to distribute oxygen, nitrous oxide, medical air, and vacuum. The pipelines' outlets act as self-closing sockets, each specifically configured, coloured, and labelled for one gas. Oxygen, nitrous oxide, and air are delivered to the anaesthetic room at a pressure of 400 kilopascals (kPa) (4 bar, 60 pounds per square inch (psi)). The gases (and vacuum) reach the anaesthetic machine via flexible reinforced hoses, colour coded throughout their length (oxygen—white, nitrous oxide—blue, vacuum—yellow). These attach to the wall outlet via a gas-specific probe (Fig. 2.7) and to the anaesthetic machine via a gas-specific nut and union. Cylinders, the traditional method of supplying

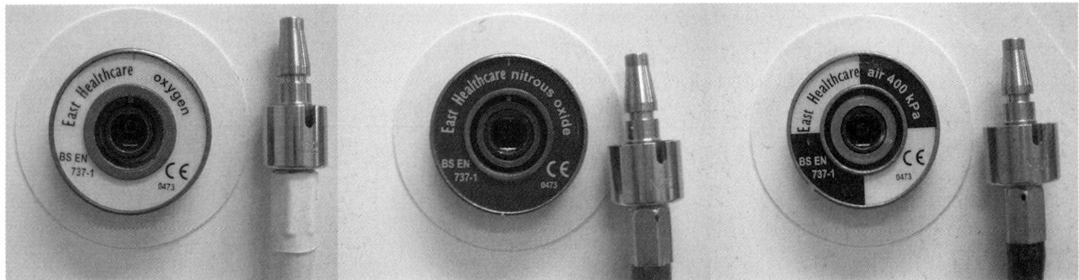

Figure 2.7 Wall-mounted outlets and gas-specific probes for (left to right) oxygen, nitrous oxide, and air.

Table 2.1 Medical gas cylinder colours.

Gas	Colour Body	Shoulder
Oxygen	Black	White
Nitrous oxide	Blue	Blue
Entonox	Blue	Blue/white
Air	Grey	White/black
Carbon dioxide	Grey	Grey

gases to the anaesthetic machine, are now mainly used as reserves in case of pipeline failure. Cylinders are also colour coded to indicate their contents (Table 2.1). Increasingly, small oxygen cylinders used during transfer of patients are all white, resulting from a move to agree white cylinder bodies for all medical gases, with the colour of the shoulder denoting the gas inside.

Oxygen

Piped oxygen is supplied from a liquid oxygen reserve, where it is stored under pressure (10–12 bar, 1200 kPa) at approximately –180°C in a vacuum-insulated evaporator (VIE), effectively a large thermos flask. Gaseous oxygen is removed from above the liquid or, at times of increased demand, by vaporizing liquid oxygen using heat from the environment. The gas is warmed to ambient air temperature en route from the VIE to the pipeline system. A reserve bank of cylinders of compressed oxygen is kept adjacent in case the main system fails. A smaller cylinder is attached directly to the anaesthetic machine as an emergency reserve. The pressure in a full cylinder is 12 000 kPa (120 bar, 1980 psi), and this falls proportionately as the cylinder empties.

Nitrous oxide

Piped nitrous oxide is supplied from several large cylinders joined together to form a bank and attached to a common manifold. There are usually two banks, one running with all cylinders turned on (duty bank), and a reserve. In addition, there is a small emergency supply. Smaller cylinders are attached directly to the anaesthetic machine. At room temperature, nitrous oxide is a liquid within the cylinder, and, while any liquid remains, the pressure within the cylinder remains constant at 5400 kPa (54 bar, 800 psi). When all the liquid has evaporated, the cylinder contains only gas and, as it empties, the pressure falls to zero.

Medical air

This is supplied either by a compressor or in cylinders. A compressor delivers air to a central reservoir, where it is dried and filtered to achieve the desired quality before distribution. Air is supplied to the operating theatre at 400 kPa for anaesthetic use, and at 700 kPa to power medical tools.

Vacuum

The final part of the PMGV system is a medical vacuum. Two pumps are connected to a system that must be capable of generating a vacuum of at least 400 mmHg below atmospheric pressure. This is delivered to the anaesthetic rooms, operating theatres, and other appropriate sites. At several stages between the outlets and the pumps there are drains and bacterial filters to prevent contamination by aspirated fluids.

The anaesthetic machine

Its main functions are to:

- reduce the high pressure gases from either the pipeline or cylinders to a pressure that is safe for onward delivery to the patient;
- control the flow of gases allowing a known, accurate, and adjustable composition to be delivered into the anaesthetic system breathing system.

In addition to these functions, many modern anaesthetic machines contain integral monitoring equipment and ventilators.

Reduction of pressure

Cylinders contain gases at very high pressures (see above) which can vary depending on the content or temperature of the cylinder. The gas from them first passes through reducing valves to ensure that a constant supply of gas at 400 kPa is delivered to the flow meters. As piped gases are already delivered at 400 kPa, no further pressure reduction is required.

Control of flow of gases

Traditionally, on most anaesthetic machines this has been achieved by the use of flowmeters ('rotameters'; Fig. 2.8):

- A specific, calibrated flowmeter is used for each gas.
- A needle valve controls the flow of gas through the flowmeter.
- Where accurate, low flows are required, two tubes are used in series: the first has a smaller diameter and a narrow, low flow range (e.g. 0–0.5 L/min), the second is wider with a greater flow range (0.5–10 L/min).
- A rotating bobbin floats in the gas stream, its upper edge indicating the rate of gas flow.
- Several flowmeters for different gases (oxygen, air, and nitrous oxide) are mounted with oxygen to the left; the control for oxygen has a different knurled finish and is usually more prominent.
- Flowmeters do not regulate pressure

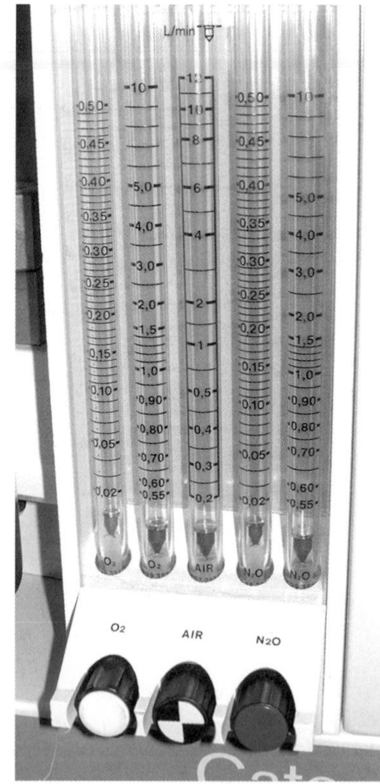

Figure 2.8 Oxygen, air, and nitrous oxide flowmeters on an anaesthetic machine.

Modern anaesthetic machines have several safety features built into the gas delivery system:

- The oxygen and nitrous oxide controls are linked, preventing <25% oxygen from being delivered.
- An emergency oxygen 'flush' device can be used to deliver pure oxygen into the breathing system.
- An audible alarm to warn of failure of oxygen delivery. This discontinues the nitrous oxide supply and, if the patient is breathing spontaneously, air can be entrained.
- A non-return valve to minimize the effects of back-pressure on the function of flowmeters and vaporizers.

Increasingly, on many modern anaesthetic machines, flowmeters have been replaced with electronic control of gas flow. The anaesthetist simply dials in the required flow and this is delivered into the anaesthetic system. The flow of gas is then displayed on a monitor screen either numerically or as an analogue representation of a flowmeter.

The addition of anaesthetic vapours

This is achieved by the use of vaporizers, devices that produce a very accurate concentration of each inhalational anaesthetic drug (Fig. 2.9).

- Vaporizers produce a saturated vapour from a reservoir of liquid anaesthetic.
- The final concentration of anaesthetic is controlled by varying the proportion of gas passing into the vapour chamber.
- The vaporizers are temperature compensated to account for the loss of latent heat that causes cooling of the liquid and a reduction in vaporization of the anaesthetic.
- Most anaesthetic machines allow more than one vaporizer to be fitted at any time. To prevent more than one vapour being given, an interlock device is fitted. This is usually a mechanical device that prevents more than one vaporizer being turned on simultaneously.

The resultant mixture of gases and vapour is finally delivered to a common outlet on the anaesthetic machine. From this point, specialized breathing systems are used to transfer the gases and vapours either to the patient or to the ventilator.

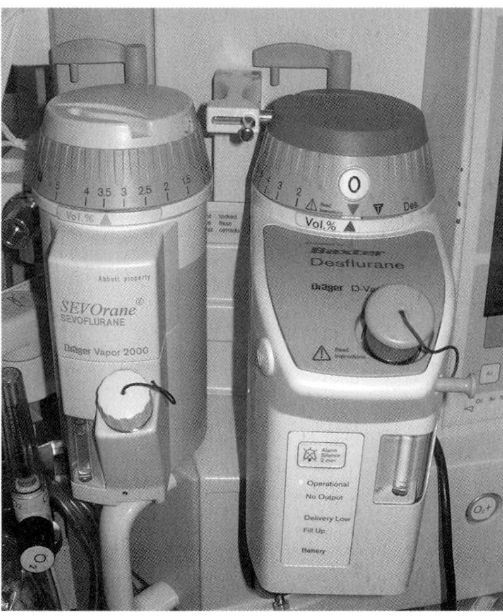

Figure 2.9 Sevoflurane vaporizer (left) and desflurane vaporizer (right) on an anaesthetic machine. Note that the interlock is positioned to prevent desflurane being given at the same time as sevoflurane.

Anaesthetic breathing systems

The mixture of anaesthetic gas and vapour travels from the anaesthetic machine to the patient via an anaesthetic circuit, or, more correctly, an anaesthetic breathing system, and finally to the patient's airway via a facemask, laryngeal mask, or tracheal tube. There are a number of different breathing systems (referred to as 'Mapleson A, B, C, D, or E') plus a circle system. The details of these systems are beyond the scope of this book, but they all have a number of common features, described below. As several patients in succession may breathe through the same system, a low-resistance, disposable bacterial filter is placed at the patient end of the system, and changed between each patient to reduce the risk of cross-infection. Alternatively, disposable systems can be used, which are changed between each patient.

Components of a breathing system

All systems consist of the following:

- *A connection for fresh gas input*: usually the common gas outlet on the anaesthetic machine.
- *A reservoir bag*: usually of 2 L capacity to allow the patient's peak inspiratory demands (30–40 L/min) to be met with a lower constant flow from the anaesthetic machine. It allows manual ventilation of the patient if needed, in a patient breathing spontaneously it gives an indication of ventilation, and it acts as a further safety device, being easily distended at low pressure if obstruction occurs.
- *An adjustable expiratory valve*: to vent expired gas, helping to eliminate carbon dioxide. During spontaneous ventilation, resistance to opening is

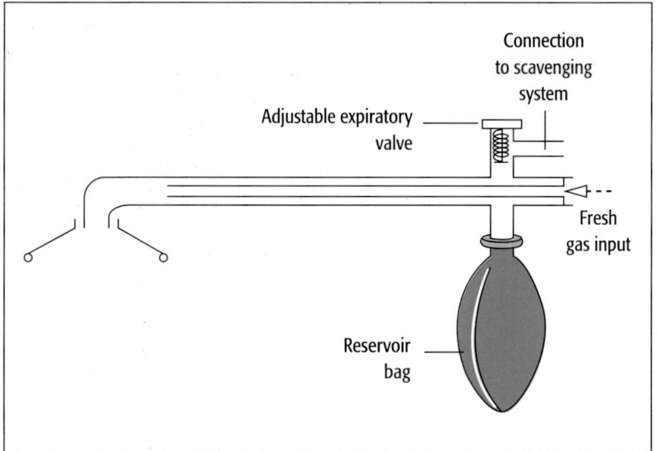

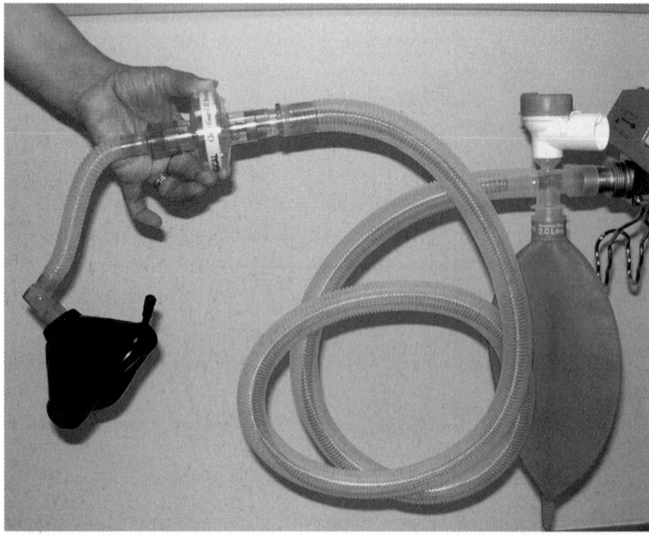

Figure 2.10 The component parts of a breathing system and photograph of the system connected to the common gas outlet on the anaesthetic machine. Note the port on the expiratory valve (white) to allow connection to the anaesthetic gas-scavenging system.

minimal so as not to impede expiration. Closing the valve allows manual ventilation by squeezing the reservoir bag.

Traditionally, circuits consisted of a length of wide-bore tubing along which the anaesthetic gases flowed to the patient. Excess and expired gases were vented into the atmosphere close to the patient. They relied on the positioning of the components of the breathing system and the gas flow from the anaesthetic machine to eliminate expired gas containing carbon dioxide, thereby preventing rebreathing and hypercapnia. Even the most efficient of these systems is still wasteful; a gas flow of 4–6 L/min is required, as expired gas also contains oxygen and anaesthetic vapour which are lost to the environment. Subsequent developments in design allowed the waste gases to be collected or 'scavenged' and deposited outside the operating environment (see below). An example of a commonly used system is shown in Fig. 2.10.

The circle system

The circle system (Fig. 2.11) overcomes many of the inefficiencies of the systems described above by 'recycling' some of the expired gas mixture.

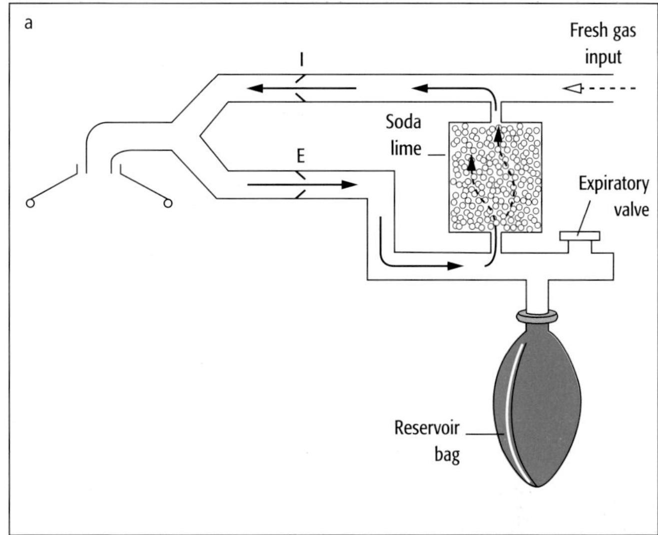

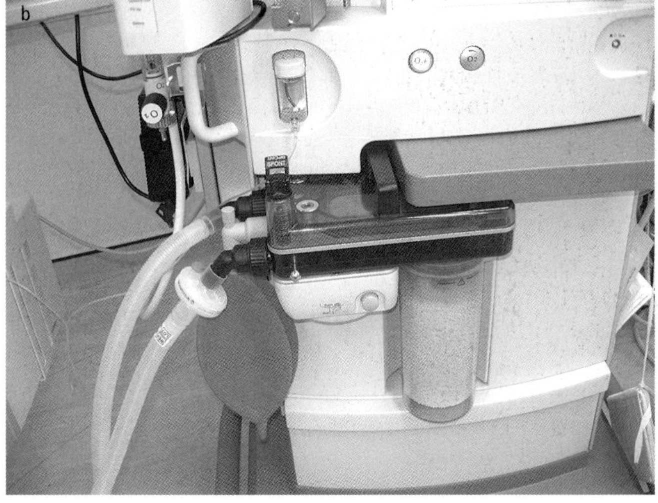

Figure 2.11 (a) Diagrammatic representation of a circle system (I, inspiratory; E, expiratory one-way valves). (b) Circle system on an anaesthesia machine. Most components are integrated; only the inspiratory and expiratory tubing, the reservoir bag, and soda lime container are obvious.

- The expired gases are passed through a container of soda lime (the absorber), a mixture of calcium, sodium, and potassium hydroxide that removes carbon dioxide chemically.
- After the carbon dioxide has been removed, the expired gas has supplementary oxygen and anaesthetic vapour added to maintain the desired concentrations, and the mixture is rebreathed by the patient.
- The gases are warmed and humidified as they pass through the absorber (a consequence of the reaction that removes carbon dioxide).

As a result, gas flows from the anaesthetic machine can be as low as 0.3–0.5 L/min. The circle system is therefore becoming increasingly popular because of the rising cost of anaesthetic inhalational drugs and the recognition of the potential polluting effects.

There are several points to note when using a circle system.

- As the inspired gas is a mixture of expired and fresh gas, the concentration of oxygen within the circle is not accurately known. The inspired oxygen concentration must be monitored to ensure that the patient is not rendered hypoxic.

- The inspired anaesthetic concentration must be monitored, particularly when a patient is being ventilated through a circle, to prevent awareness.
- An indicator is incorporated into the soda lime so that when it is unable to absorb any more carbon dioxide the granules change colour. One of the commonly used preparations changes from pink to white.

Patients can breathe spontaneously or be ventilated via both of the systems described above.

Mechanical ventilation

A wide variety of anaesthetic ventilators are available, each of which functions in a slightly different way. An outline of the principles of mechanical ventilation is given, and the interested reader should consult 'Further reading' at the end of the chapter.

During spontaneous ventilation, a negative intrathoracic pressure is generated, causing gas to move into the lungs. This process is reversed during mechanical ventilation. A positive pressure is applied to the anaesthetic gases to overcome airway resistance and elastic recoil of the chest causing gas flow into the lungs. This technique is usually referred to as *intermittent positive pressure ventilation* (IPPV). In order to generate the positive pressure, the ventilator requires a source of energy: generally gas pressure or electricity. In both spontaneous and mechanical ventilation, expiration occurs by passive recoil of the lungs and chest wall.

Gas pressure

Gas from the anaesthetic machine collects in a bellows, or bag, situated in a rigid container. The ventilator controls the delivery of a gas (usually oxygen) at high pressure into the container to compress the bellows or bag, delivering the contents to the patient. This system is often called a 'bag-in-bottle' ventilator.

Electricity

Electrical power opens and closes valves to control the flow (and volume) of gas from a high-pressure source. Alternatively, an electric motor can power a piston within a cylinder to deliver a volume of gas to the patient. Modern ventilators increasingly rely on complex electronics to control gas delivery, and the inspiratory and expiratory timing of ventilation.

The modern anaesthetic machine

Advances in technology have allowed virtually all of the above functions to be integrated into a single unit (Fig. 2.12). Electronic controls (Fig. 2.13) then allow the anaesthetist to determine:

- spontaneous or controlled ventilation;
- the flow of each gas required;
- the inspired oxygen concentration.

If mechanical ventilation is being used, the following can be controlled:

- tidal volume;
- respiratory rate;
- the mode of ventilation, usually a choice between volume and pressure controlled (see Chapter 6);
- the inspiratory and expiratory times;
- peak inspiratory pressure;
- the use of positive end expiratory pressure.

Some machines allow the vapour concentration to be set; on others the concentration from the vapourizer is set and adjusted to achieve the required end-tidal concentration. All of the above are monitored and displayed, and can be set to alarm if they fall outside predetermined limits. In case of power failure there is a back-up battery supply to maintain key operations, and if this fails the patient can still be ventilated manually.

Minimizing theatre pollution

Unless special measures are taken, the atmosphere in the operating theatre will become polluted with anaesthetic gases. The breathing systems described and mechanical ventilators vent varying volumes of excess and expired gas into the atmosphere, the patient expires anaesthetic gas during recovery, and there are leaks from anaesthetic apparatus. Although no conclusive evidence exists to link

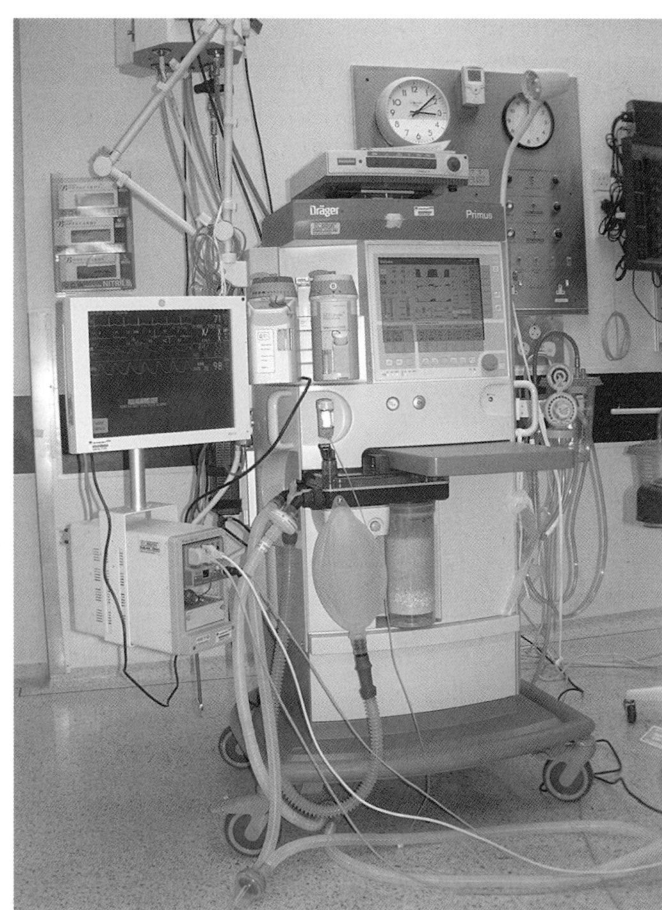

Figure 2.12 Modern integrated anaesthesia machine and monitors.

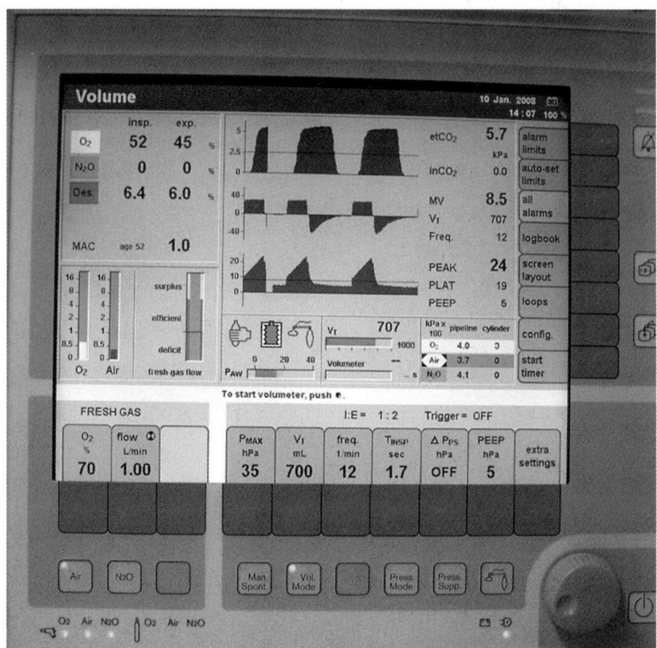

Figure 2.13 Close-up of controls and display of monitoring on the anaesthesia machine shown in Fig. 2.12.

prolonged exposure to low concentrations of inhalational anaesthetics with any risks, it would seem sensible to minimize the degree of pollution within the operating theatre environment. This can be achieved in a number of ways:

- reducing the flow of gases, for example by use of a circle system;
- avoiding the use of gases, for example by use of total intravenous anaesthesia (TIVA), regional anaesthesia;
- using air conditioning in the theatre;
- scavenging systems.

Scavenging systems

These collect the gas vented from breathing systems and ventilators and deliver it via a pipeline system to the external atmosphere. The most widely used is an active system in which a small negative pressure is applied to the expiratory valve of the breathing system or ventilator to remove gases to the outside environment. The patient is protected against excessive negative pressure being applied to the lungs by valves with very low opening pressures. The use of such systems does not eliminate the problem of pollution; it merely shifts it from one site to another; both nitrous oxide and, to a lesser extent, the inhalational anaesthetics are potent destroyers of ozone, thereby adding to the greenhouse effect.

Measurement and monitoring

Measurement and monitoring are closely linked but are not synonymous. A measuring instrument becomes a monitor if it is capable of delivering a warning when the variable being measured falls outside preset limits. During anaesthesia, both the patient and the equipment being used are monitored.

Monitoring the patient

Monitoring of the ECG, blood pressure (non-invasive), pulse oximetry, capnometry, and oxygen and vapour concentrations is now regarded as essential for the safe conduct of anaesthesia. Various other parameters may also be monitored depending on the patient and the operation.

The ECG

This is easily applied and gives information on heart rate and rhythm; it may indicate the presence of ischaemia and acute disturbances of certain electrolytes (e.g. potassium and calcium). It can be monitored using three leads: one applied to the right shoulder (red), another to the left shoulder (yellow) and a third to the left lower chest (green), which will give a tracing equivalent to standard lead II of the 12-lead ECG. Many ECG monitors now use five electrodes placed on the anterior chest to allow all the standard leads and V5 to be displayed. The ECG alone gives no information on the adequacy of the cardiac output, and it must be remembered that it is possible to have a virtually normal ECG with minimal cardiac output.

Non-invasive blood pressure

This is the most common method of monitoring the patient's blood pressure during anaesthesia and surgery. Auscultation of the Korotkoff sounds is difficult in the operating theatre, and so automated devices are widely used. A cuff, commonly placed around the arm over the brachial artery, is inflated by an electrical pump. The cuff then undergoes controlled deflation. A microprocessor-controlled pressure transducer detects variations in cuff pressure resulting from transmitted arterial pulsations. Initial pulsations represent systolic blood pressure, and peak amplitude of the pulsations equates to mean arterial pressure. Diastolic is then calculated using an algorithm.

Heart rate is also determined and displayed. The pneumatic cuff must have a width that is *40% of the arm circumference*, and the internal inflatable bladder should encircle at least half the arm. If the cuff is too small, the blood pressure will be overestimated, and if it is too large it will be underestimated. The frequency of blood pressure estimation can be set, and the monitor can be set to alarm if the recorded blood pressure falls outside predetermined limits. Such devices cannot measure pressure continually, and become increasingly inaccurate at extremes of pressure and in patients with an arrhythmia.

Pulse oximeter

A probe, containing a light-emitting diode (LED) and a photodetector, is applied across the tip of a digit or earlobe. The LED emits red light, alternating between two different wavelengths in the visible and infrared regions of the electromagnetic spectrum. These are transmitted through the tissues and absorbed to different degrees by the tissues, oxyhaemoglobin, and deoxyhaemoglobin. The intensity of light reaching the photodetector is converted to an electrical signal. Absorption by the tissues is constant, but absorption by blood varies with the cardiac cycle; this allows determination of the peripheral arterial oxygen saturation (SpO_2), both as a waveform and as a digital reading.

Pulse oximeters are accurate to ±2%. The waveform can also be interpreted to give a reading of the heart rate. Alarms can be set for levels of saturation and heart rate. Therefore, the pulse oximeter gives information about both the circulatory and respiratory systems and has the advantages of:

- providing continuous monitoring of oxygenation at tissue level;
- being unaffected by skin pigmentation;
- portability (mains or battery powered);
- being non-invasive.

Despite this, there a number of important limitations of this device:

- There is failure to appreciate the severity of hypoxia; a saturation of 90% equates to a PaO_2 of 8 kPa (60 mmHg) because of the shape of the haemoglobin dissociation curve.
- It is unreliable when there is severe vasoconstriction due to the reduced pulsatile component of the signal.
- It is unreliable with certain haemoglobins:
  - carboxyhaemoglobin; results in overestimation of SpO_2;
  - methaemoglobinaemia; at an SaO_2 >85%, results in underestimation of the saturation.
- It progressively under-reads the saturation as the haemoglobin falls (but it is not affected by polycythaemia).
- It is affected by extraneous light.
- It is unreliable when there is excessive movement of the patient.
- The pulse oximeter is not an indicator of the adequacy of alveolar ventilation as hypoventilation can be compensated for by increasing the inspired oxygen concentration to maintain oxygen saturation.

In many modern anaesthesia systems, the above monitors are integrated and displayed on a single screen (Fig. 2.14).

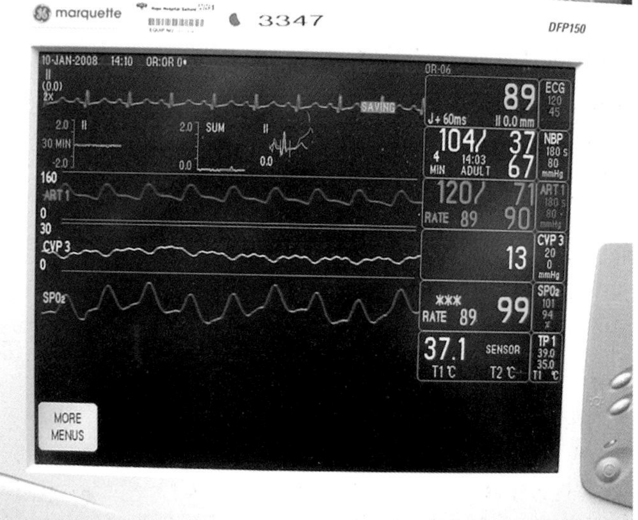

Figure 2.14 Integrated monitoring system displaying: ECG and heart rate (beats/min), non-invasive blood pressure (mmHg), arterial waveform and invasive blood pressure, cental venous pressure (CVP) and waveform, pulse oximeter waveform and saturation (SpO_2), and temperature.

Capnometry

The capnometer (often referred to as a capnograph) works on the principle that carbon dioxide (CO_2) absorbs infrared light in proportion to its concentration. In a healthy person, the CO_2 concentration in alveolar gas (or partial pressure, $PaCO_2$) correlates well with the partial pressure in arterial blood ($PaCO_2$), the former being lower, by 5 mmHg or 0.7 kPa. Analysis of gas in the breathing system at the end of expiration (i.e. *end-tidal CO_2* concentration) reflects $PaCO_2$. Capnometry is primarily used as an indicator of the adequacy of ventilation; $PaCO_2$ is inversely proportional to alveolar ventilation. In patients with a low cardiac output (e.g. hypovolaemia, PE), the gap between arterial and end-tidal CO_2 increases (end-tidal falls), mainly due to the development of increased areas of ventilation/perfusion mismatch. The gap also increases in patients with chest disease due to poor mixing of respiratory gases. Care must be taken in interpreting end-tidal CO_2 concentrations in these circumstances. Modern capnometers have alarms for when the end-tidal CO_2 is outside preset limits. Other uses of capnometry are given in Table 2.2.

Vapour concentration analysis

Whenever a volatile anaesthetic is given, the concentration in the inspired gas mixture should be monitored. This is usually achieved using infrared absorption, similarly to CO_2. The degree of absorption is dependent specifically on the volatile and its concentration. A single device can be calibrated for all of the commonly used inhalational anaesthetics.

Peripheral nerve stimulator

This is used to assess neuromuscular blockade after giving neuromuscular blocking drugs, for example at the end of surgery to see if there is any residual block that needs reversing. A peripheral nerve supplying a discrete muscle group is stimulated transcutaneously with a current of 50 mA. The resulting contractions are observed or measured. One arrangement is to stimulate the ulnar nerve at the wrist whilst monitoring the contractions (twitch) of the adductor pollicis. Although most often done by looking at or feeling the response, measuring either the force of contraction or the compound action potential is more objective. Sequences of stimulation used include:

- four stimuli each of 0.2 s duration, at 2 Hz for 2 s, referred to as a 'train-of-four' (TOF);
- one stimulus at 50 Hz of 5 s duration, i.e. a tetanic stimulus;
- two groups of three tetanic bursts at 50 Hz, 750 ms apart.

During non-depolarizing neuromuscular blockade, there is a *progressive* decremental response to all the sequences, termed 'fade'. In the TOF, the ratio of the amplitude of the fourth twitch (T4) to the first twitch (T1) is used as an index of the degree of

Table 2.2 Uses of capnometry.

- An indicator of the degree of alveolar ventilation:
  - to ensure normocapnia during mechanical ventilation
  - to control the level of hypocapnia in neurosurgery
  - avoidance of hypocapnia where the cerebral circulation is impaired, e.g. the elderly
- As a disconnection indicator (the reading suddenly falls to zero)
- To indicate that the tracheal tube is in the trachea (CO_2 in expired gas)
- As an indicator of the degree of rebreathing (presence of CO_2 in inspired gas)
- As an indicator of cardiac output. If cardiac output falls and ventilation is maintained, then end-tidal CO_2 falls as CO_2 is not delivered to the lungs, e.g.
  - hypovolaemia
  - cardiac arrest, where it can also be used to indicate effectiveness of external cardiac compression
  - massive pulmonary embolus
- It may be the first clue of the development of malignant hyperpyrexia

neuromuscular blockade. The absence of any response is either seen with profound neuromuscular block, for example shortly after a drug has been given, or is the result of failure to deliver a stimulus. During depolarizing blockade, the response to all sequences of stimulation is reduced but consistent, i.e. there is no fade.

Temperature

During anaesthesia the patient's temperature is usually continually monitored. The most commonly used device is a thermistor, a semiconductor that varies in resistance according to its temperature. This can be placed in the oesophagus (cardiac temperature) or nasopharynx (brain temperature). The rectum can be used but, apart from being unpleasant, faeces may insulate the thermistor, leading to inaccuracies. An infrared tympanic membrane thermometer can be used intermittently, but the external auditory canal must be clear. Although temperature is normally measured to help identify and prevent hypothermia, a sudden unexpected rise in a patient's temperature may be the first warning of the development of MH (see page 84).

Invasive or direct blood pressure

This is the most accurate method for measuring and monitoring blood pressure, and is generally reserved for use in complex, prolonged surgery or sick patients. A cannula is inserted into a peripheral artery and connected via a fluid-filled tube to a transducer that converts the pressure signal into an electrical signal. This is then amplified and displayed as both a waveform and blood pressure (see Fig. 2.14).

Central venous pressure (CVP)

This is measured by inserting a catheter via a central vein, usually the internal jugular or subclavian, so that its tip lies at the junction of the superior vena cava and right atrium. It is then connected as described above to display a waveform and pressure (Fig. 2.14).

Although absolute values of the CVP can be measured, its trend is usually more informative. Often a 'fluid challenge' is used in the face of a low CVP (see page 114). The CVP is measured, a rapid infusion of fluid is given, and the change in CVP noted. In the hypovolaemic patient the CVP increases briefly and then falls back to around the previous value, whereas in the euvolaemic patient the CVP will show a greater and more sustained rise. Overtransfusion will be seen as a high, sustained CVP.

CVP is usually monitored during operations in which there is the potential for major fluid shifts or blood loss, or for those patients in whom even small fluid shifts may be detrimental, for example heart failure. It is affected by a variety of other factors apart from fluid balance (Table 2.3), in particular cardiac function. Hypotension in the presence of an elevated CVP (absolute or in response to a fluid challenge) may indicate heart failure. However, most clinicians would now accept that monitoring left ventricular function with either transoesophageal Doppler or a pulmonary artery flotation catheter (page 134) is preferable.

Blood loss

Strictly speaking, this is measured rather than monitored. Simple estimates of blood loss during surgery are easily performed. Swabs can be weighed, dry and wet, the increase in weight giving an indication of the amount of blood they have absorbed. The volume of blood in the suction apparatus can

Table 2.3 Factors affecting the central venous pressure.

- The zero reference point
- Patient posture
- Fluid status
- Heart failure
- Raised intrathoracic pressure:
  - mechanical ventilation
  - coughing
  - straining
- Pulmonary embolism
- Pulmonary hypertension
- Tricuspid valve disease
- Pericardial effusion, tamponade
- Superior vena cava obstruction

be measured, with allowance for irrigation fluids. Such methods are only estimates, as blood may remain in body cavities, or be spilt on the floor and absorbed by drapes and gowns. In paediatric practice, where small volumes of blood loss are relatively more important, all absorbent materials are washed to remove the blood and the resultant solvent analysed by colorimetry to estimate blood loss.

Many other physiological parameters can be, and are, measured during anaesthesia when appropriate. Some examples are: clotting profiles and haemoglobin concentration in patients receiving a transfusion of a large volume of stored blood; blood glucose in diabetic patients; and arterial blood gas and acid–base analysis during the bypass phase of cardiac surgery. Recently, interest has been shown in the development of monitors that give information relating to the depth of anaesthesia, but these are still under investigation.

It is essential to recognize that the above standards apply not only to those patients undergoing general anaesthesia, but also to those receiving sedation, local or regional anaesthesia, and during transfer.

Finally, one should never rely solely on monitors—regular observation and examination of the patient and clinical judgement are essential to avoid acting on false information.

Monitoring the equipment

With the increasing reliance on complex equipment to deliver anaesthesia, the AAGBI recommends that there should be continuous monitoring of the continuity of the oxygen supply and correct functioning of the breathing system.

Oxygen supply

All anaesthetic machines are fitted with a device warning of oxygen supply failure. Continuous monitoring of the oxygen concentration in the inspired gas mixture is considered essential. This is usually achieved using a fuel cell oxygen analyser that produces a current proportional to the oxygen concentration, displayed as a numeric value of oxygen concentration. *It must be remembered that the inspired oxygen concentration does not guarantee adequate arterial oxygen saturation* as it may be insufficient to compensate for the effects of hypoventilation and ventilation/perfusion mismatch (see page 90).

Breathing systems

Irrespective of whether the patient is breathing spontaneously or being ventilated, capnometry will alert the anaesthetist to most of the common problems, for example disconnection (loss of reading), inadequate gas flow (increased *end-tidal* CO_2), or hyper/hypoventilation (decreased/increased *end-tidal* CO_2, respectively). In addition, when a patient is mechanically ventilated, airway pressures must be monitored to avoid excessive pressures being generated within the lungs. Airway pressure monitoring can also be used as a secondary indicator of inadequate ventilation in ventilated patients; high pressures may be the result of obstruction (e.g. blocked tracheal tube, bronchospasm), and loss of pressure may be the result of a disconnection. The latter function may be specifically used as a 'disconnection alarm'.

Drugs and fluids used during anaesthesia

Anaesthetists have to be familiar with a wide range of drugs, obviously those directly associated with anaesthesia, but also those taken by patients for other medical conditions that may impact upon anaesthesia. Furthermore, unlike in most other branches of medicine, drugs associated with anaesthesia are almost always given parenterally: either IV or via inhalation, and often have undesirable actions in addition to their intended effects on the central nervous system (CNS). As well as drugs, many patients will also require IV fluids, blood, and blood products during anaesthesia and surgery, and postoperatively.

Premedication

This refers to the administration of any drugs in the period before induction of anaesthesia, in addition to those normally taken by the patient. The aims of premedication are summarized in Table 2.4.

Anxiolysis

The most commonly prescribed drugs for this are the benzodiazepines. They are well absorbed from the gastrointestinal tract, produce a degree of sedation and amnesia, and are usually given orally 45–90 min preoperatively. Those most commonly used include temazepam 20–30 mg, diazepam 10–20 mg, and lorazepam 2–4 mg. Beta-blockers may be given to patients who suffer from excessive somatic manifestations of anxiety, for example tachycardia. A preoperative visit for explanation and reassurance is often as effective as any drug at alleviating anxiety, and sedation does not always mean lack of anxiety.

Amnesia

Some patients specifically request that they do not have any recall of the events leading up to anaesthesia and surgery. This may be accomplished by the administration of lorazepam (as above) to provide anterograde amnesia.

Table 2.4 The six As of premedication.

- Anxiolysis
- Amnesia
- Antiemetic
- Antacid
- Antiautonomic
- Analgesia

Antiemetic (reduction of nausea and vomiting)

These drugs are often given as a premed to try and reduce the incidence of PONV. The incidence of PONV is increased when opioids are given intraoperatively, after certain types of surgery, for example gynaecology, ear, nose, and throat (ENT), and urology, and in female patients. Unfortunately, none of the currently used drugs can be relied on totally to prevent or treat established PONV. Combination therapy is most effective. Drugs with antiemetic properties are shown in Table 2.5.

Antacid (modify pH and volume of gastric contents)

Patients are starved preoperatively to reduce the risk of regurgitation and aspiration of gastric acid at the induction of anaesthesia (see below). This may not be possible or effective in some patients, for example:

- those who require emergency surgery;
- those who have received opiates or are in pain will show a significant delay in gastric emptying;
- those with a hiatus hernia, who are at an increased risk of regurgitation.

A variety of drug combinations are used to try and increase the pH and reduce the volume of gastric contents.

- *Ranitidine (H_2 antagonist)*: 150 mg orally 12 hourly and 2 hourly preoperatively.
- *Omeprazole (proton pump inhibitor)*: 40 mg 3–4 hourly preoperatively.
- *Metoclopramide*: 10 mg orally preoperatively. Both increases gastric emptying and lowers oesophageal sphincter tone. Often given in conjunction with ranitidine.

Table 2.5 Commonly used antiemetic drugs, dose, and route of administration.

Type of drug	Example	Usual dose
Dopamine antagonists	Metoclopramide	10 mg orally or IV
5-Hydroxytryptamine antagonists	Ondansetron	4–8 mg orally or IV
Antihistamines	Cyclizine	50 mg IM or IV
Anticholinergics	Hyoscine	1 mg transdermal patch

- *Oral sodium citrate (0.3 M)*: 30 mL orally to chemically neutralize residual acid. Most commonly used immediately before induction of anaesthesia for caesarean section.

If a naso- or orogastric tube is in place, this can be used to aspirate gastric contents.

Antiautonomic effects

Anticholinergic effects

- Reduce salivation (antisialogogue), for example during fibreoptic intubation, surgery, or instrumentation of the oral cavity, or ketamine anaesthesia.
- Reduce the vagolytic effects on the heart, for example before the use of suxamethonium (particularly in children), during surgery on the extra ocular muscles (squint correction), or during elevation of a fractured zygoma.

Atropine and hyoscine have now largely been replaced preoperatively by glycopyrrolate, 0.2–0.4 mg intramuscularly (IM). Many anaesthetists would consider an IV dose given at induction more effective.

Antisympathomimetic effects

Intubation increases sympathetic activity, causing tachycardia and hypertension. This is undesirable in certain patients, for example those with ischaemic heart disease or raised intracranial pressure. These responses can be attenuated by giving beta-blockers orally as part of the premed (e.g. atenolol, 25–50 mg) or IV at induction (e.g. esmolol). Perioperative beta-blockade may also decrease the incidence of adverse coronary events in high-risk patients undergoing major surgery. An alternative is to give a potent analgesic at induction of anaesthesia, for example fentanyl, alfentanil, or remifentanil.

Analgesia

Although the sedative effect of morphine is the oldest form of premedication, analgesic drugs are now generally given to patients who are in pain preoperatively. The most commonly used are morphine and fentanyl. Opiates have a range of unwanted side-effects, including nausea, vomiting, respiratory depression, and delayed gastric emptying.

Miscellaneous

A variety of other drugs are commonly given prophylactically before anaesthesia and surgery, for example:

- *steroids*: to patients on long-term treatment, or who have received them within the past 3 months;
- *antibiotics*: to patients with prosthetic or diseased heart valves, undergoing joint replacement or bowel surgery;
- *anticoagulants*: as prophylaxis against DVT;
- *transdermal glyceryl trinitrate (GTN)*: as patches for patients with ischaemic heart disease to reduce the risk of coronary ischaemia;
- *eutectic mixture of local anaesthetics (EMLA)*: a topically applied local anaesthetic cream to reduce the pain of inserting an IV cannula.

> The majority of the patient's own regular medications should be taken as normal, unless instructed otherwise by the anaesthetist.

Intravenous anaesthetic drugs

This group of drugs is most commonly used to induce anaesthesia. After IV injection, these drugs are carried in the bloodstream into the cerebral circulation. As they are very lipid soluble, they quickly cross the blood–brain barrier, resulting in loss of consciousness. Subsequently the drug is rapidly redistributed to other tissues (initially the muscles and then fat), and so the plasma and brain concentrations fall and the patient recovers consciousness. A single bolus of these drugs has a rapid onset, short duration of action, with rapid recovery. Despite this, complete elimination of some drugs, usually by hepatic metabolism, takes much longer, and repeated doses may lead to accumulation and delayed recovery. This is seen typically with thiopentone, and currently the only exception to this is propofol (see below). All these drugs cause depression of the cardiovascular and respiratory systems. The dose required to induce anaesthesia is significantly reduced in those patients who are elderly, frail, hypovolaemic, or have compromise of their cardiovascular system.

A synopsis of the drugs commonly used is given in Table 2.6.

Inhaled anaesthetic drugs

These drugs are most commonly used to maintain anaesthesia, although they can also be used to induce anaesthesia. They are halogenated hydrocarbons with relatively low boiling points, so they evaporate easily at ambient temperature and the resulting vapour is breathed by the patient; hence they are often referred to as vapours. The vapour reaches the patient's lungs either as a result of spontaneous respiratory effort or via a ventilator. Once in the lungs they diffuse into the blood in the pulmonary capillaries and are then distributed via the systemic circulation to the brain and other tissues. It is the partial pressure of these drugs in the brain that is responsible for the anaesthetic effect, and this is closely related to the partial pressure in the alveoli. The rate at which the alveolar partial pressure can be changed determines the rate of change in the brain and hence the speed of induction, and change in depth of, and recovery from, anaesthesia. However, even the most rapid induction using these drugs takes several minutes to achieve the same depth of anaesthesia that is achieved within seconds of giving an IV anaesthetic drug. Nitrous oxide is the only other drug in this category. The inspired concentration of all of these compounds is expressed as the percentage by volume. All the inhalational anaesthetics cause dose-dependent depression of the cardiovascular and respiratory systems. A synopsis of the drugs used is given in Table 2.7.

There are two concepts that will help in understanding the use of inhalational anaesthetics: solubility and minimum alveolar concentration.

Solubility

One of the main determinants of alveolar partial pressure is how soluble the inhalational anaesthetic is in blood. Relatively *insoluble* anaesthetics (e.g. sevoflurane, desflurane) diffuse slowly from the alveoli into the pulmonary blood. As little anaesthetic is removed from the alveoli, the partial pressure rises quickly, followed by a similarly rapid rise in blood and brain partial pressure, and anaesthesia is induced rapidly. In contrast, a *soluble* anaesthetic (e.g. halothane) diffuses rapidly from the alveoli into the pulmonary blood, limiting the rate of rise of alveolar and brain partial pressure. Consequently, induction will be slower. Recovery from anaesthesia follows similar principles in reverse. Only a small amount of an insoluble drug will have to be excreted to allow the partial pressure within the brain to fall. A larger amount of a more soluble drug will need to be excreted to achieve the same effect, which will take proportionately longer.

Other factors that determine the speed at which the alveolar concentration rises include:

- *A high inspired concentration*: limited clinically by the degree of irritation caused by the vapour.
- *Alveolar ventilation*: this is most pronounced for drugs with a high solubility. As large amounts are removed from the alveoli, increasing ventilation ensures more rapid replacement.
- *Cardiac output*: if high, results in a greater pulmonary blood flow, increasing uptake and thereby lowering the alveolar partial pressure. If low, the converse occurs and the alveolar concentration rises more rapidly.

Minimum alveolar concentration

To compare the potencies and side-effects of the inhalational anaesthetics, the concept of *minimum alveolar concentration* (MAC) is used. This is the concentration required to prevent movement following a surgical stimulus in 50% of subjects. At 1 MAC, or multiples thereof, the anaesthetic effect will be the same and a comparison of the side-effects can be made. Compounds with a low potency (e.g. desflurane) will have a high MAC; those with a high potency (e.g. isoflurane) will have a low MAC.

The effects of inhalational anaesthetics are additive; therefore two values for MAC are often quoted—the value in oxygen and the value when

Table 2.6 Intravenous drugs used for the induction of anaesthesia and their effects.

Drug	Induction dose (mg/kg)	Speed of Induction (s)	Duration of action (min)	Effects on CVS	Effects on RS	Effects on CNS	Other side-effects	Comments
Propofol	1.5–2.5	30–45	4–7	Hypotension, worse if hypovolaemic or cardiac disease	Apnoea up to 60 s, depression of ventilation	Decreases CBF and ICP	Pain on injection, involuntary movement, hiccoughs	Non-cumulative, repeated injections or infusion used to maintain anaesthesia (see TIVA)
Etomidate	0.2–0.3	30–40	3–6	Relatively less cardiovascular depression	Depression of ventilation	Decreases CBF and ICP, anticonvulsant	Pain on injection, involuntary movement, hiccoughs	Emulsion available, less painful. No histamine release, non-cumulative, but suppresses steroid synthesis
Thiopentone	2–6	20–30	9–10	Dose-dependent hypotension, worse if hypovolaemic or cardiac disease	Apnoea, depression of ventilation	Decreases CBF and ICP, anticonvulsant	Rare but severe adverse reactions	Patients may 'taste' garlic or onions! Cumulative, delayed recovery after repeat doses
Ketamine	1–2	50–70	10–12	Minimal in fit patients, better tolerated if cardiovascular compromise	Minimal depression of ventilation, laryngeal reflexes better preserved, bronchodilation	CBF maintained, profound analgesia	Vivid hallucinations	Subanaesthetic doses cause analgesia. Can be used as sole anaesthetic drug in adverse circumstances, e.g. prehospital
Midazolam	0.1–0.3	40–70	10–15	Dose-dependent hypotension, worse if hypovolaemic or cardiac disease	Depression of ventilation, worse in elderly	Mildly anticonvulsant		Causes amnesia

CVS, cardiovascular system; RS, respiratory system; CNS, central nervous system; CBF, cerebral blood flow; ICP, intracranial pressure; TIVA, total intravenous anaesthesia.

Table 2.7 Inhalational anaesthetic drugs and their effects.

Compound	Potency	Solubility	Effect on CVS	Effect on RS	Effect on CNS	Comments
Sevoflurane	Low: 6–7% for induction, 2–3% for maintenance	Low: rapid changes of depth	↓BP, vasodilatation	Depresses ventilation	Minimal effect on CBF at clinical concentration	Popular for inhalation induction
Desflurane	Low: 6–9% for maintenance	Low; rapid changes of depth	↓BP, ↑HR	Depresses ventilation	Minimal effect on CBF at clinical concentration	Pungent, boils at 23°C
Isoflurane	Medium; 5% for induction, 1–1.5% for maintenance	Medium	↓BP, ↑HR, vasodilatation	Depresses ventilation	Slight ↑CBF and ICP	Pungency limits use for induction
Halothane	High: 3–4% for induction, 0.5–1% for maintenance	High	↓BP, vasodilatation, myocardial depression, arrhythmias common	Depresses ventilation	↑↑CBF, ↑ICP	May cause hepatitis on repeat exposure
Enflurane	Medium: 1.5–2% for maintenance	Medium	↓BP	Depresses ventilation	↑CBF, ↑EEG activity	Pungency limits use for induction

CVS, cardiovascular system; RS, respiratory system; CNS, central nervous system; BP, blood pressure; HR, heart rate; CBF, cerebral blood flow; ICP, intracranial pressure; EEG, electroencephalograph.

Table 2.8 MAC values for inhalational anaesthetics.

	Sevoflurane (%)	Desflurane (%)	Isoflurane (%)	Halothane (%)	Enflurane (%)
In 100% oxygen	2.2	6.0	1.3	0.75	1.6
In 70% nitrous oxide	1.2	2.8	0.6	0.3	0.6

given with a stated percentage of nitrous oxide (which has its own MAC), which will clearly be less (Table 2.8).

The value of MAC is reduced in the elderly, in those with hypotension, hypothermia, and hypothyroidism, and with concurrent use of opioids; it is increased in infants, patients with a pyrexia, and in those who are chronic drug abusers.

Nitrous oxide

Nitrous oxide (N_2O) is a colourless, sweet-smelling, non-irritant vapour with moderate analgesic properties but low anaesthetic potency (MAC 105%). The maximum safe inspired concentration that can be administered without the risk of causing hypoxia is approximately 70%; therefore, unconsciousness or anaesthesia sufficient to allow surgery is rarely achieved. Consequently, it is usually given in conjunction with one of the other vapours. Nitrous oxide is available in cylinders premixed with oxygen as a 50:50 mixture called 'Entonox' which is used as an analgesic in obstetrics and by the emergency services.

Systemic effects

- Cardiovascular depression, worse in patients with pre-existing cardiac disease.
- A slight increase in the respiratory rate and a decrease in the tidal volume. It decreases the ventilatory response to hypercarbia and hypoxia.
- Cerebral vasodilatation, increasing intracranial pressure (ICP).
- Diffuses into air-filled cavities more rapidly than nitrogen can escape, causing either a rise in pressure (e.g. in the middle ear) or an increase in volume (e.g. within the gut or an air embolus).
- May cause bone-marrow suppression by inhibiting the production of factors necessary for the synthesis of DNA. The length of exposure necessary may be as short as a few hours, and recovery usually occurs within 1 week.
- At the end of anaesthesia, nitrous oxide rapidly diffuses into the alveoli reducing the partial pressure of oxygen, and can result in hypoxia (diffusion hypoxia) if the patient is breathing air. This can be overcome by increasing the inspired oxygen concentration during recovery from anaesthesia.

Total intravenous anaesthesia

When IV drugs alone are given to induce and maintain anaesthesia, the term 'total intravenous anaesthesia' (TIVA) is used. For a drug to be of use in maintaining anaesthesia, it must be rapidly metabolized to inactive substances or eliminated to prevent accumulation and delayed recovery, and have no unpleasant side-effects. Currently, an infusion of propofol is the most widely used technique; ketamine is associated with an unpleasant recovery, etomidate suppresses steroid synthesis, and recovery after barbiturates is prolonged due to their accumulation.

Neuromuscular blocking drugs

These work by preventing acetylcholine interacting with the postsynaptic (nicotinic) receptors on the motor end plate on the muscle membrane (and possibly other sites). Muscle relaxants are divided into two groups and named to reflect what is thought to be their mode of action.

Depolarizing neuromuscular blocking drugs

Suxamethonium

This is the only drug of this type in regular clinical use. It comes ready prepared (50 mg/mL, 2 mL ampoules). The dose in adults is 1.5 mg/kg IV. After injection, there is a short period of muscle fasciculation as the muscle membrane is depolarized, followed by muscular paralysis in 40–60 s. Recovery occurs spontaneously as suxamethonium is hydrolysed by the enzyme plasma (pseudo-) cholinesterase, and normal neuromuscular transmission is restored after 4–6 min. This rapid onset makes it the drug of choice to facilitate tracheal intubation in patients likely to regurgitate and aspirate.

Suxamethonium has no direct effect on the cardiovascular, respiratory, or central nervous systems. Bradycardia secondary to vagal stimulation is common after very large or repeated doses, and can be avoided by pretreatment with atropine. Suxamethonium has a number of important side-effects (Table 2.9).

Pseudocholinesterase deficiency

A variety of genes have been identified which are involved in pseudocholinesterase production. The most significant genotypes are:

- normal homozygotes: sufficient enzyme to hydrolyse suxamethonium in 4–6 min (950 per 1000 population);
- atypical heterozygotes: slightly reduced enzyme levels; suxamethonium lasts 10–20 min (50 per 1000);
- atypical homozygotes: marked deficiency of enzyme; members of this group remain apnoeic for up to 2 h after being given suxamethonium (<1 per 1000).

Treatment of a patient found to have severe deficiency of pseudocholinesterase is with maintenance of anaesthesia or sedation and ventilatory support until spontaneous recovery occurs. The patient should subsequently be warned and given a card that carries details and, because of its inherited nature, the remainder of the family should be investigated.

Non-depolarizing neuromuscular blocking drugs

These drugs compete with acetylcholine and block its access to the postsynaptic receptor sites on the muscle, but do not cause depolarization. (They may also block presynaptic receptors responsible for facilitating the release of acetylcholine.) They are sometimes referred to as competitive neuromuscular blockers. The time to maximum effect, i.e. when relaxation is adequate to allow tracheal intubation, is relatively slow compared with suxamethonium, generally 1.5–3 min. A synopsis of the drugs used is given in Table 2.10.

They are used in two ways:

- following suxamethonium to maintain muscle relaxation during surgery;
- to facilitate tracheal intubation in non-urgent situations.

Although recovery of normal neuromuscular function will eventually occur spontaneously after the use of these drugs, it is often accelerated by the administration of an anticholinesterase (see below).

Anticholinesterases

The action of all the neuromuscular blocking drugs will wear off spontaneously with time, but this is

Table 2.9 Important side-effects of suxamethonium.

- Malignant hyperpyrexia in susceptible patients
- Increased intraocular pressure which may cause loss of vitreous in penetrating eye injuries
- Muscular pain around the limb girdles, most common 24 h after administration in young adults
- Histamine release: usually localized but may cause an anaphylactic reaction
- Prolonged apnoea in patients with pseudocholinesterase deficiency (see below).
- A massive rise in serum potassium may provoke dysrhythmias in patients with:
  - burns, maximal 3 weeks to 3 months after the burn
  - denervation injury, e.g. spinal cord trauma, maximal after 1 week
  - muscle dystrophies, for example Duchenne's
  - crush injury

Table 2.10 Non-depolarizing neuromuscular blocking drugs.

Drug	Dose for intubation	Maintenance dose	Time to intubation	Duration of action	Systemic effects	Comments
Atracurium	0.5–0.6 mg/kg	0.15–0.2 mg/kg; 30–50 mg/h infusion	90–120 s	20–25 min	Cutaneous histamine release, ↓BP	Spontaneous degradation in plasma. Cisatracurium a single isomer, more potent
Rocuronium	0.6–0.7 mg/kg	0.15–0.2 mg/kg; 30–50 mg/h infusion	90–100 s; after 1 mg/kg, 60 s	20–30 min	Minimal	Alternative to suxamethonium for RSI
Vecuronium	0.1 mg/kg	0.02–0.03 mg/kg; 6–10 mg/h infusion	90–120 s	15–20 min	Minimal, no histamine release	White powder, dissolved before use
Mivacurium	0.15–0.2 mg/kg	0.1 mg/kg	100–120 s	10–15 min	Histamine released if large dose injected rapidly	Metabolized by plasma cholinesterase. Rapid recovery, reversal often unnecessary
Pancuronium	0.1 mg/kg	0.015 mg/kg	120–150 s	35–45 min	↑BP, ↑HR	Long acting

BP, blood pressure; HR, heart rate; RSI, rapid-sequence induction.

not always clinically appropriate or convenient. If reversal of neuromuscular blockade is required, an anticholinesterase is given. This inhibits the action of the enzyme acetylcholinesterase, leading to an increase in the concentration of acetylcholine within the synaptic cleft of the neuromuscular junction. The speed of recovery will depend upon the intensity of block when reversal is attempted—the more intense the block, the slower the reversal. Anticholinesterases cannot be used to reverse a very intense block, for example if given soon after the administration of a relaxant (no response to a TOF sequence—see above).

Anticholinesterases also increase the amount of acetylcholine within parasympathetic synapses (muscarinic receptors), causing bradycardia, spasm of the bowel, bladder, and bronchi, increased bronchial secretions, etc. To prevent these unwanted muscarinic effects, they are always administered with a suitable dose of atropine or glycopyrrolate.

The most commonly used anticholinesterase is neostigmine:

- A fixed dose of 2.5 mg IV is used in adults.
- Its maximal effect is seen after approximately 5 min and lasts for 20–30 min.
- It is given concurrently with either atropine 1.2 mg or glycopyrrolate 0.5 mg.

Sugammadex

This is a newly developed drug that appears able to reverse even an intense neuromuscular block induced by neuromuscular blocking drugs of the aminosteroid group, rocuronium and vecuronium. Using sugammadex removes the need for, and unwanted side-effects of, both anticholinesterases and anticholinergics when reversing residual neuromuscular block. Sugammadex appears to be otherwise inactive, with no effects on acetylcholinesterase or any other receptors. It is currently undergoing final clinical safety trials.

Analgesic drugs

Analgesic drugs are used as part of the anaesthetic technique to eliminate pain, reduce the autonomic response to surgery, and allow lower concentrations of inhalational or IV drugs to be given to maintain anaesthesia.

Opioid analgesics

This term is used to describe all drugs that have an analgesic effect mediated through opioid receptors, including both naturally occurring and synthetic compounds. The term 'opiate' is reserved for naturally occurring substances, for example morphine. They produce their effects at a cellular level by activating opioid receptors. These receptors are distributed throughout the CNS, in particular in the substantia gelatinosa of the spinal cord and the peri-aqueductal grey matter of the mid-brain. There are several types of opioid receptors, and since their identification they have had a variety of names. The current nomenclature for identification of opioid receptors is that approved by the International Union of Pharmacology: MOP, KOP, and DOP (mu, kappa, and delta opioid peptide) receptors, each of which has a number of different subtypes. Opioid analgesics can have pure agonist, partial agonist, or mixed (agonist and antagonist) actions at the receptors.

Pure agonists

This group of drugs produces the classical effects of opioids: analgesia, euphoria, sedation, depression of ventilation, and physical dependence. The systemic effects of opioids are due to both central and peripheral actions, and are summarized in Table 2.11.

A synopsis of the pure agonists used in anaesthesia is given in Table 2.12. Because of the potential for physical dependence, there are strict rules laid out in the Misuse of Drugs Act 1971 which govern the issue and use of most opioid drugs (see below).

Tramadol

A weak agonist predominantly at MOP receptors with approximately 10% of morphine's potency, but all of the side-effects, for example nausea, vomiting, and constipation. Tramadol also blocks the reuptake of noradrenaline and 5-hydroxytryptamine (5-HT) within the CNS, thereby augmenting descending inhibitory pathways that modulate pain perception. As a result, naloxone can only reverse the MOP receptor-mediated actions, provid-

Table 2.11 Central and peripheral actions of opioids.

Central nervous system	Respiratory system	Gastrointestinal tract
Analgesia	Antitussive effect	Reduced peristalsis causing:
Sedation	Bronchospasm in susceptible patients	• constipation
Euphoria	**Cardiovascular system**	• delayed gastric emptying
Nausea and vomiting	Peripheral venodilatation	Constriction of sphincters
Pupillary constriction	Bradycardia due to vagal stimulation	**Endocrine system**
Depression of ventilation:	**Skin**	Release of ADH and
• rate more than depth	Itching	catecholamines
• reduced response to CO_2		
Depression of vasomotor centre		
Addiction (not with normal clinical use)		
Urinary tract		
Increased sphincter tone and urinary retention		

ADH, antidiuretic hormone.

Table 2.12 The pure opioid agonists used in anaesthesia.

Drug	Route given	Dose	Speed of onset	Duration of action (min)	Comments
Morphine	IM	0.2–0.3 mg/kg	20–30 min	60–120	Also given subcutaneously, rectally, epidurally, intrathecally
	IV	0.1–0.15 mg/kg	5–10 min	45–60	Effective against visceral pain and pain of myocardial ischaemia Less effective in trauma
Fentanyl	IV	1–3 μg/kg	2–3 min	20–30	Short procedures, spontaneous ventilation
		5–10 μg/kg	1–2 min	30–60	Long procedures, controlled ventilation
Alfentanil	IV	10 μg/kg	30–60 s	5–10	Short procedures. May cause profound respiratory depression
	IV infusion	0.5–2 μg/kg/min	30–60 s	Infusion dependent	Long procedures, controlled ventilation
Remifentanil	IV infusion	0.1–0.3 μg/kg/min	15–30 s	Infusion dependent	Major procedures. Very rapid recovery. Profound respiratory depression. Widely used in TIVA
Pethidine	IM	1–2 mg/kg	15–20 min	30–60	Marked nausea and vomiting. Less effect on smooth muscle

TIVA, total intravenous anaesthesia.

ing only partial reversal. Well absorbed orally, the dose is 50–100 mg not more frequently than 4 hourly. Similar doses can be given IV or IM.

The partial agonists and mixed agonists/antagonists

These drugs were introduced in the hope that, with only partial agonist activity or mixed agonist/antagonist actions, analgesia would be achieved without the problem of depression of ventilation. Such an ideal has not yet been achieved.

Nalbuphine, meptazinol, and pentazocine

These are synthetic analgesics that have agonist actions at one opioid receptor and antagonist actions at another receptor. Nalbuphine is similar in potency and duration of action to morphine, and exhibits a ceiling effect of analgesia. Meptazinol has only one-tenth the potency of morphine and a high incidence of nausea and vomiting. Pentazocine has about one-quarter the potency of morphine.

Buprenorphine

This is a partial agonist, but 30 times more potent than morphine, with a longer duration of action, up to 8 h. It is well absorbed when given sublingually. Nausea and vomiting may be severe and prolonged. Not completely reversed by naloxone (see below).

The pure antagonist

The only one in common clinical use is naloxone. This has antagonist actions at all the opioid receptors, reversing all the centrally mediated effects of pure opioid agonists.

- The initial IV dose in adults is 0.1–0.4 mg, effective in less than 60 s and lasts 30–45 min.
- It has a limited effect against opioids, with partial or mixed actions, and complete reversal may require very high (10 mg) doses.
- Following a severe overdose of opioids, either accidental or deliberate, several doses or an infusion of naloxone may be required, as its duration of action is shorter than that of most opioids.

- Interestingly, naloxone also reverses the analgesia produced by acupuncture, suggesting that this is probably mediated in part by the release of endogenous opioids.

The regulation of opioid drugs

Some drugs have the potential for abuse and cause physical dependence, and their use in medicine is carefully regulated. The Misuse of Drugs Act 1971 relates to 'dangerous or otherwise harmful drugs', which are designated 'Controlled Drugs', and include the opioids. The Act attempts to prevent the misuse of these substances by imposing a total prohibition on their manufacture, possession, and supply. The Misuse of Drugs Regulations 2001 permits the use of Controlled Drugs in medicine. The drugs covered by these regulations are classified into five schedules, each subject to a different level of control.

Schedule 1 Hallucinogenic drugs, including cannabis and lysergic acid diethylamide (LSD), which currently have no recognized therapeutic use.

Schedule 2 This includes opioids, major stimulants (amphetamines and cocaine), and secobarbital.

Schedule 3 Drugs thought less likely to be misused than those in schedule 2, and includes barbiturates, minor stimulants, buprenorphine, and temazepam.

Schedule 4 This is split into two parts:

- benzodiazepines (except temazepam), which are recognized as having the potential for abuse;
- androgenic steroids, clenbuterol, and growth hormones.

Schedule 5 Preparations which contain very low concentrations of codeine or morphine, for example cough mixtures.

Supply and custody of schedule 2 drugs

In the operating theatre complex, these drugs are supplied by the pharmacy, usually at the signed, written request of a senior member of the nursing staff, specifying the drug and total quantity required. These drugs must be stored in a locked safe, cabinet, or room, constructed and maintained in a way that prevents unauthorized access. A record must be kept of their use in the 'Controlled Drugs Register' and must comply with the following requirements:

- Separate parts of the register can be used for different drugs or strengths of drugs within a single class.
- The class of drug must be recorded at the head of each page.
- Entries must be in chronological sequence.
- Entries must be made on the day of the transaction or the next day.
- Entries must be in ink or otherwise indelible.
- No cancellation, alteration, or obliteration may be made.
- Corrections must be accompanied by a dated footnote.
- The register must not be used for any other purpose.
- A separate register may be used for each department (i.e. each theatre).
- Registers must be kept for 2 years after the last dated entry.

The specific details required with respect to supply of Controlled Drugs (i.e. for the patient) are: the date of the transaction, name of person supplied (i.e. the patient's name), licence of person to be in possession (doctor's signature with name printed), amount given to the patient, and the amount, if any, from the ampoule not given and destroyed. A fresh ampoule(s) must be used for each patient.

Non-steroidal anti-inflammatory drugs (NSAIDs)

These drugs inhibit the enzyme cyclo-oxygenase (COX) and therefore prevent the synthesis of prostaglandins, prostacyclins, and thromboxane A2 from arachidonic acids. They have anti-inflammatory, analgesic, and antipyretic actions. There are two main isoenzymes of cyclo-oxygenase: COX-1 and COX-2.

- COX-1: constitutive enzyme, responsible for synthesizing prostaglandins involved in protection of the integrity of the gastric mucosa, maintenance of renal blood flow, particularly during shock, platelet aggregation to reduce bleeding, and bone healing.

• COX-2: inducible, peripherally by surgery, trauma, and endotoxins, and in the CNS by pain.

The inhibition of COX-1 produces the unwanted effects, and inhibition of COX-2 the desired therapeutic effects. The older NSAIDs are non-specific and associated with a greater incidence of complications, with elderly patients being particularly vulnerable. More recently, COX-2-specific NSAIDs have become available. These target only the inducible form of the enzyme and were originally thought to have a lower incidence of complications. Unfortunately, in long-term clinical use, this does not appear to be the case and some of these drugs have been associated with increased risk of stroke and MI. Their main role now is in the short-term management of acute pain. The relative and absolute contraindications to the use of these drugs are given in Table 2.13.

A commonly used NSAID in anaesthesia is parecoxib.

• A selective COX-2 inhibitor, with predominantly analgesic activity, usually given IV, but can be given IM.

• Initial IV dose 40 mg, subsequent doses 20–40 mg, 6–12 hourly, maximum 80 mg/day for 2 days. Reduce dose by 50% in elderly.

• Effective after orthopaedic surgery; has opioid-sparing effects after abdominal surgery.

• No effect on ventilation or cardiovascular function.

• Not subject to the Misuse of Drugs Regulations.

Paracetamol

An analgesic and antipyretic with little anti-inflammatory action, but usually classified with NSAIDs. It inhibits prostaglandin synthesis, mainly in the CNS. It is well absorbed when taken orally, with minimal adverse effect on the gastrointestinal tract. Widely used orally for the treatment of mild to moderate pain in a dose of 1 g 4–6 hourly, maximum 4 g/day, and is often incorporated into compound preparations with aspirin or codeine. An IV preparation is available containing 10 mg/mL, in 100 mL vials (1 g). The dose is the same as for the oral preparation, can be infused over 15 min, and is effective in 5–10 min. It is the safest of all analgesics, but patients may need reassurance that regular dosing of 1 g every 6 h is not associated with hepatic toxicity.

Local anaesthetic drugs

When applied to nervous tissue, these drugs cause a reversible loss of the ability to conduct nerve impulses. They can be given by a variety of routes, including topically, subcutaneously, or directly adjacent to nerves.

Table 2.13 Relative and absolute contraindications to the use of NSAIDs in anaesthesia.

Relative contraindications	Absolute contraindications
High risk of intraoperative bleeding, e.g. vascular surgery	Pre-existing renal dysfunction, hyperkalaemia
Concurrent use of ACE inhibitors, anticoagulants, nephrotoxic drugs	Cardiac failure
Hepatic dysfunction	Severe hepatic dysfunction
Bleeding disorders	History of GI bleeding
Elderly (>65 years)	Hypersensitivity to NSAIDs
Pregnancy and during lactation	Aspirin-induced asthma
Asthma	

ACE, angiotensin-converting enzyme; GI, gastrointestinal; NSAIDs, non-steroidal anti-inflammatory drugs.

Mechanism of action

At rest, a nerve cell has a transmembrane electrical potential (voltage) of –70 mV, and is said to be polarized. Noxious, mechanical, thermal, or chemical stimuli, depending on their intensity, allow sodium ions (Na^+) to enter the cell. If the stimulus is of sufficient intensity, a depolarization threshold is reached that triggers another type of sodium channel (voltage-gated) to open. As a result, the cell's membrane potential increases to +20 mV and an 'action potential' is initiated. This local change in the cell's membrane electrical potential causes adjacent voltage-gated sodium channels to open, altering that segment's membrane potential, propagating the action potential along the nerve. The membrane is rapidly repolarized to the resting level by loss of potassium ions (K^+) from within the cell, followed by active pumping out of Na^+ in exchange for K^+ by the Na/K pump. During repolarization, no action potential can be propagated by that section of nerve, thus ensuring unidirectional travel of action potentials. Not all stimuli are sufficient to reach the threshold, and so some will not lead to an action potential being initiated or propagated. Action potentials are 'all or nothing' events, and all of equal magnitude. Consequently, the strength of a nervous impulse is solely dependent on the frequency of action potentials.

In myelinated nerves, the rate of conduction is vastly increased as the action potential 'jumps' between the nodes of Ranvier, a process known as 'saltatory conduction'.

Local anaesthetic drugs work by blocking the sodium channels from within the nerve cell, preventing entry of sodium and subsequent depolarization so that no action potentials can be initiated or propagated.

Local anaesthetic drugs exist in two forms: ionized and unionized. When a local anaesthetic is given, the majority will exist as the ionized form but, in order to cross the cell membrane, it has to be in the unionized form. This change occurs after injection because of a relatively higher pH in tissues (7.4 compared with 6.0 in solution). However, the intracellular pH is lower (7.1) and so a greater proportion returns to its ionized form. It is this form that is attracted to, and then blocks, the sodium channels. Clearly, the degree of unionized drug will have an effect on the speed of onset. This can be further increased by using a higher concentration of the drug.

The duration of action will be determined by what proportion is protein bound; generally, the greater the binding to membrane proteins, the longer the duration of action. Local blood supply will also have an effect as this will affect the speed of removal of the drug. The degree of lipid solubility will determine potency by influencing the membrane penetration by the drug, but will also result in a tendency for greater toxicity.

Following the injection of a local anaesthetic drug, there is always a predictable sequence to the onset of effects as small diameter nerves are blocked before large diameter ones, and unmyelinated nerves are blocked before myelinated ones. Consequently when a regional anaesthetic technique is used, the order of onset of the block is:

- Autonomic fibres—vasodilatation
- Temperature
- Pain
- Touch
- Motor—paralysis

This accounts for the warm feeling that patients frequently notice at the onset of spinal or epidural anaesthesia, and the fact that under some circumstances patients feel no pain but can still move their legs.

Individual drugs

Local anaesthetic drugs can be divided into two groups on the basis of their chemical structure:

- Esters: amethocaine, benzocaine, cocaine
- Amides: lignocaine, bupivacaine, prilocaine

The esters were the first drugs to be introduced into clinical practice. They are relatively more toxic, allergenic, and unstable than their modern counterparts the amides. Their main use today is to provide topical anaesthesia.

Amethocaine

Available as a 4% gel (Ametop) that is applied topically at the site of intended IV cannulation, and is effective in 45 min. More dilute solutions are available to provide topical anaesthesia of the conjunctiva.

Cocaine

Available as a paste and spray in concentrations of 4–10%. Its main use is to provide topical anaesthesia of the nasal cavity, with the added advantage that its profound vasoconstrictor (sympathomimetic) properties reduce bleeding. This effect is also responsible for its toxicity and risk of arrhythmias.

Lignocaine

A commonly used local anaesthetic in a variety of techniques including topically, by infiltration, nerve blocks, and epidural and spinal anaesthesia. Consequently it is available in a range of concentrations, 0.5–10%, to suit all situations. It is often combined with adrenaline (see below). It has a relatively fast onset and medium duration of effect. The currently accepted maximum safe dose is:

- 3 mg/kg, maximum 200 mg (without adrenaline)
- 6 mg/kg, maximum 500 mg (with adrenaline)

These doses should be reduced if the patient is elderly, frail, or shocked. It can also be used in the treatment of VF/VT refractory to defibrillation (100 mg IV) when amiodarone is unavailable. As with all amide local anaesthetics, it is metabolized in the liver.

Bupivacaine

Bupivacine has a slower onset but a greater duration of action than lignocaine, and is widely used for nerve blocks, and epidural and spinal anaesthesia, particularly in obstetric anaesthesia. It is available as either 0.25 or 0.5% solutions, with or without adrenaline, and as 0.1 and 0.125% solutions that are used for epidural infusion to provide pain relief during labour. The current maximum safe dose is 2 mg/kg, with or without adrenaline, in any 4 h period. Bupivacaine is significantly more cardiotoxic than other amide local anaesthetics, and toxicity is difficult to treat (see below).

Bupivacaine molecules can exist in two forms that are 'mirror images' of each other, termed stereoisomers. The solution used clinically is a racemic mixture, meaning it contains both forms in equal quantities. The two different forms of the molecule are described according to various conventions, the most commonly used being based upon their ability to rotate polarized light, either; + or D (dextrorotatory), – or L (laevorotatory). Recently, levobupivacaine (Chirocaine) has been introduced into clinical practice. As its name suggests, this is the pure L-form of the molecule. The dose used is the same as for bupivacaine, but its main advantage is significantly reduced card iotoxicity.

Prilocaine

Closely related to lignocaine, its advantage is a reduced toxicity for a given dose. Its main use now is infiltration anaesthesia in dental surgery, when high concentrations are used. It is also a component of EMLA, a *e*utectic *m*ixture of *l*ocal *a*naesthetics. This is a cream that contains lignocaine and prilocaine in equal proportions (25 mg of each per gram). It is applied to the skin and produces surface analgesia in approximately 60 min. It is used to reduce the pain associated with venepuncture in children.

A synopsis of the drugs used for local and regional anaesthesia is given in Table 2.14.

Adrenaline (epinephrine)

Adrenaline is a potent vasoconstrictor as a result of its action at alpha-adrenergic receptors and is added to local anaesthetics to reduce blood flow at the site of injection. This has several beneficial effects, notably to reduce the rate of absorption, reduce toxicity, and extend the duration of action. This is most effective during infiltration anaesthesia and nerve blocks, and less effective in epidurals or spinals. Some authorities recommend that solutions containing adrenaline should never be used intrathecally. Only very small concentrations of adrenaline are required to obtain intense vasoconstriction. The concentration is expressed as the weight of adrenaline (g) per volume of solution

Table 2.14 Local anaesthetic drugs.

Drug	Dose	Speed of onset	Duration of action	Comments
Lignocaine	3 mg/kg (plain), max. 200 mg 6 mg/kg (with adrenaline), max. 500 mg	Rapid	60–180 min, depending on the technique used	Used: topically, infiltration, nerve blocks, IVRA, epidurally, intrathecally
Bupivacaine	2 mg/kg, max. 150 mg	Nerve block: up to 40 min	Up to 24 h	Mainly used for nerve blocks, epidurally and intrathecally.
	(±adrenaline) in any 4 h period	Epidurally: 15–20 min	3–4 h, dose dependent	Relatively cardiotoxic
		Intrathecal: 30 s	2–3 h, dose dependent	
Levobupivacaine	An isomer of bupivacaine; most properties very similar, but less cardiotoxic. This allows slightly higher doses to be given			
Ropivacaine	3 mg/kg, max. 200 mg	Similar to bupivacaine	For the same concentration and technique, shorter than bupivacaine	At lower concentrations, relatively less intense motor block than bupivacaine

IVRA, intravenous regional anaesthesia.

(mL). Commonly used concentrations range from 1:80 000 to 1: 200 000.

Local anaesthetics containing vasoconstrictors are not used around extremities (e.g. fingers, toes, penis), because of the risk of vasoconstriction causing tissue necrosis.

The maximum safe dose of adrenaline in an adult is 250 μg, i.e. 20 mL of 1:80 000 or 50 mL of 1:200 000. This should be reduced by 50% in patients with ischaemic heart disease.

Calculation of doses

For any drug, it is essential that the correct dose is given and that the maximum safe dose is never exceeded. This can be confusing with local anaesthetic drugs as the volume containing the required dose will vary depending upon the concentration (expressed in per cent), and a range of concentrations exists for each drug. The relationship between concentration, volume, and dose is given by the formula:

$$\text{Concentration (\%)} \times \text{Volume (mL)} \times 10 = \text{dose (mg)}$$

Intravenous fluids

During anaesthesia fluids are given IV to replace losses due to surgery, and to provide the patient's normal daily requirements. Three types are used: crystalloids, colloids, and blood and its components.

Crystalloids

These are solutions of crystalline solids in water. The solutions can be considered in two groups: those that contain electrolytes in a similar composition to plasma, have an osmolality similar to plasma, and are often referred to as being isotonic; and those that contain less or no electrolytes (hypotonic) but contain glucose to ensure that they have an osmolality similar to plasma. A summary of the composition of the most commonly used crystalloids is shown in Table 2.15. Once these fluids are given, they are redistributed amongst the various body fluid compartments, the extent depending on their composition. For example, 0.9% saline is distributed throughout the intravascular and interstitial volumes (extracellular fluid (ECF)

Table 2.15 Composition of crystalloids.

Crystalloid	Na^+ (mmol/L)	K^+ (mmol/L)	Ca^{2+} (mmol/L)	Cl^- (mmol/L)	HCO_3^- (mmol/L)	pH	Osmolality (mosmol/L)
Hartmann's	131	5	4	112	29*	6.5	281
0.9% sodium chloride	154	0	0	154	0	5.5	300
4% glucose + 0.18% sodium chloride	31	0	0	31	0	4.5	284
5% glucose	0	0	0	0	0	4.1	278

*Present as lactate which is metabolized to bicarbonate by the liver.

compartment) in proportion to their size. After 15–30 min, only 25–30% of the volume administered remains intravascular. Therefore, if such a fluid is used to restore the circulating volume, three to four times the deficit will need to be given. If a hypotonic solution is given, for example 5% glucose, once the glucose is metabolized the remaining fluid is distributed throughout the entire body water (i.e. ECF and intracellular fluid (ICF) volumes), and less than 10% will remain intravascular. Saline (0.9%) and Hartmann's solution are widely used in the perioperative period and as the first line for emergency fluid resuscitation. However, large volumes may cause hyperchloraemic metabolic acidosis, as, although regarded as isotonic, they both contain a greater concentration of chloride than plasma. Glucose-containing solutions are a way of treating dehydration as a result of water losses but may cause hyponatraemia. They are not routinely used perioperatively.

Recently interest has been shown in the use of hypertonic saline, consisting of between 1.8 and 7.5% sodium chloride solutions. When given, these raise the osmolality of the ECF (mainly the intravascular component) and create a gradient such that water moves from the ICF into the plasma. The intravascular volume is expanded by a greater volume than the volume of hypertonic solution given; for example, 250 mL of 7.5% saline results in plasma expansion by up to 1.5 L. However, if given repeatedly, they will result in intracellular dehydration. Their main use at present is in resuscitation.

Colloids

These are suspensions of high molecular weight particles. The most commonly used are derived from gelatin (Haemaccel®, Gelofusine®), protein (albumin), or starch (HAES-steril®). Colloids primarily expand the intravascular volume and can initially be given in a volume similar to the estimated deficit to maintain the circulating volume. However, they have a finite life in the plasma and will eventually be either metabolized or excreted, and therefore need replacing. A summary of their composition is shown in Table 2.16. All colloids have a number of side-effects; anaphylaxis with the gelatins, and coagulopathy and bleeding with starches. Itching may also be a problem after the use of starches. There is no limit on the volume of gelatins that can be given (provided that haemoglobin concentration is maintained!) whereas starches are limited to 30–50 mL/kg.

Table 2.16 Composition of colloids.

Colloid	Average mol. wt (kDa)	Na^+ (mmol/L)	K^+ (mmol/L)	Ca^{2+} (mmol/L)	Cl^- (mmol/L)	HCO_3^- (mmol/L)	pH	Osmolality (mosmol/L)
Haemaccel	35	145	5	6.2	145	0	7.3	350
Gelofusine	35	154	0.4	0.4	125	0	7.4	465
Albumin	69	130–160	2	0	120	0	6.7–7.3	270–300
Starch	140–400	154	0	0	154	0	5.5	310

Blood and blood components

Before use, donated whole blood is generally processed into the following products to allow the most appropriate components to be given.

- *Red cells in optimal additive solution (SAG-M)* A red cell concentrate to which a mixture of saline, adenine, and glucose and mannitol has been added. This improves both red cell survival and flow characteristics. Each unit contains approximately 300 mL with a haematocrit of 50–70%, and will raise a patient's Hb by roughly 1 g/dL. White cells are routinely removed in the UK to prevent the risk of prion disease transmission.
- *Platelet concentrates* Supplied either as 'units' containing 50–60 mL (55×10^9 platelets) or as bags equivalent to four units. Four units or one bag will raise the platelet count by $30–40 \times 10^9$/L. These are given via a standard giving set *without* the use of a microaggregate filter, as this will result in the loss of significant numbers of platelets.
- *Fresh frozen plasma (FFP)* One unit consists of the plasma separated from a single donation, usually 200–250 mL, and frozen within 6 h. It contains normal levels of clotting factors (except factor VIII, 70% normal). An adult dose is four units. It should be infused as soon as it has thawed.
- *Cryoprecipitate* On controlled thawing of FFP a precipitate is formed, which is collected and suspended in plasma. It contains large amounts of factor VIII and fibrinogen. It is supplied as a pooled donation from six packs of FFP in one unit and must be used as soon as possible after thawing.

Risks of blood and blood product transfusions

All blood donations are routinely tested for hepatitis B surface antigen, hepatitis C, syphilis, human T-cell lymphotrophic virus (HTLV), and antibodies to HIV. However, a period exists between exposure to viruses and the development of antibodies. The resultant infected red cells would not be detected by current screening techniques. The risk is very small, and has been estimated for hepatitis B at $1:10^5$ and for HIV at $1:10^6$ units transfused.

In order to try and eliminate these risks, techniques now exist for using the patient's own blood in the perioperative period. This also has the advantage of reducing but not eliminating the wrong unit of blood being transfused.

- *Predepositing blood* Over a period of 4 weeks prior to surgery, the patient builds up a bank of 2–4 units of blood for retransfusion perioperatively.
- *Preoperative haemodilution* Following induction of anaesthesia 0.5–1.5 L of blood is removed and replaced with colloid. This can then be transfused at the end of surgery.
- *Cell savers* These devices collect blood lost during surgery via a suction system; the red cells are separated, washed, and resuspended, ready for retransfusion to the patient.

Further reading

Aitkenhead A, Rowbotham DJ, Smith G (eds). *Textbook of anaesthesia*, 4th edn. Edinburgh: Churchill Livingstone, 2001.

Al-Shaikh B, Stacey S. *Essentials of anaesthetic equipment*, 2nd edn. Edinburgh: Churchill Livingstone, 2001.

British Medical Association and the Royal Pharmaceutical Society of Great Britain. *British National Formulary (BNF)*. London: British Medical Association and the Royal Pharmaceutical Society of Great Britain. (Current issue available at BNF website: http://www.bnf.org/)

Gan TJ, Meyer T, Apfel CC *et al*., and Department of Anesthesiology, Duke University Medical Center. Consensus guidelines for managing postoperative nausea and vomiting. *Anesthesia and Analgesia* 2003; **97**: 62–71.

Gosling P. Salt of the earth or a drop in the ocean? A pathophysiological approach to fluid resuscitation. *Emergency Medicine Journal* 2003; **20**: 306–15.

Gwinnutt C, Driscoll P (eds). *Trauma resuscitation: the team approach*, 2nd edn. Oxford: BIOS Scientific, 2003.

Wildsmith JAW, Armitage EN (eds). *Principles and practice of regional anaesthesia*, 2nd edn. Edinburgh: Churchill Livingstone, 1993.

Yentis SM, Hirsch NP, Smith GB. *Anaesthesia and intensive care A to Z: an encyclopaedia of principles and practice*. Edinburgh: Butterworth Heinemann, 2003.

Useful websites

http://www.aagbi.org/
[The Association of Anaesthetists of Great Britain & Ireland.]

http://www.rcoa.ac.uk/
[The Royal College of Anaesthetists.]
These two sites are a must if you want to have the latest national UK guidance on anaesthetic practice.

http://www.frca.co.uk/
[AnaesthesiaUK. The most popular website for trainees in anaesthesia.]

http://www.theairwaysite.com/wordpress/home/devices/
[This site is aimed at emergency physicians and oriented to American practice. It does, however, contain some useful information about airway equipment.]

http://www.lmaco.com/products.php
[The laryngeal mask airway company website, which has instruction manuals for all the variations in current use. Note that several other companies now make laryngeal mask type devices.]

http://www.capnography.com/index.html
[This is an excellent site if you want to know more about capnography. Very detailed, so be warned.]

http://www.nice.org.uk/guidance/index.jsp?action=byID&r=true&o11474
[Guidance from the National Institute for Health and Clinical Excellence (NICE) on the use of ultrasound locating devices for placing central venous catheters.]

http://guidance.nice.org.uk/CG46
[Venous thromboembolism: reducing the risk of venous thromboembolism (deep vein thrombosis and pulmonary embolism) in patients undergoing surgery. NICE. April 2007.]

http://www.jr2.ox.ac.uk/bandolier/booth/painpag/
[The Oxford Pain site. Excellent for the latest evidence-based reviews in pain.]

http://www.mhra.gov.uk/
[Medicines and Healthcare products Regulatory Agency. This agency ensures that medicines, healthcare products, and medical equipment meet appropriate standards of safety, quality, performance, and effectiveness, and are used safely. The site contains the latest drug and device hazards.]

http://www.aagbi.org/publications/guidelines/docs/bloodtransfusion06.pdf
[Association of Anaesthetists guidelines on blood transfusion and component therapy, 2005.]

http://www.shotuk.org/
[Serious Hazards of Transfusion (SHOT). Contains latest UK data.]

http://www.carg.cochrane.org/en/index.html
[This site contains systematic reviews of aspects of anaesthetic practice.]

All websites last accessed April 2008.

Self-assessment

2.1 Describe briefly the physical principles of a pulse oximeter. What circumstances limit the usefulness of this device?

2.2 Describe how oxygen, nitrous oxide and medical air are stored and supplied to the operating theatres. What are the key safety characteristics of the hoses carrying these gases in the operating theatre?

2.3 Describe the sequence of pharmacological and clinical events when a dose of suxamethonium is given. Give 4–6 important side-effects.

2.4 How do non-steroidal anti-inflammatory drugs work? What are the absolute and relative contraindications to their use?

2.5 Describe how a nerve impulse is transmitted. How do local anaesthetic drugs affect this? How much lidocaine is contained in 15 ml of a 0.75% solution? What is the maximum safe dose, with and without adrenaline?

Chapter 3

The practice of anaesthesia

From the time the patient arrives in the anaesthetic room until the point they leave should follow a smooth, controlled sequence of preplanned events. This chapter aims to outline how, by applying the knowledge and skills from the previous chapter, the anaesthetist achieves this, thereby minimizing the risks of both anaesthesia and surgery. The descriptions given follow as closely as possible the sequence of events as they might be expected to occur during a normal anaesthetic.

Preoperative checks

Checking the anaesthetic machine

It is the responsibility of every anaesthetist to check that the anaesthetic machine, monitors, breathing system, and any ancillary equipment will function in the manner expected at the beginning of each operating session. The main danger is that the anaesthetic machine appears to perform normally, but in fact is delivering a hypoxic mixture to the patient. Most modern integrated anaesthesia machines perform a 'self-test' when first switched on and do not need to be re-tested by the user. A check of the gas supply, patency, and lack of gas leaks in the breathing system is essential. The function, calibration, and alarm settings on the monitors should also be checked. The AAGBI publish a document entitled *Checking Anaesthetic Equipment* that gives more comprehensive details. A record should be kept of each check of the anaesthetic machine and equipment. Appropriate procedures must also be in place to deal safely with any machine failure.

Checking the patient

The anaesthetist has a duty of care to ensure that the correct patient is anaesthetized and the correct site is operated upon. Therefore, when the patient arrives in the anaesthetic room, the anaesthetist must confirm the patient's identity, as well as the site, side (if appropriate), and nature of the planned operation. This is usually done verbally, but occasionally an unconscious patient may need surgery, for example an intensive care patient. Great care should be taken, and the patient's name-band must be checked against the notes, operating list, and consent form, preferably by both the anaesthetist and the surgeon.

Preparation for anaesthesia

Several things now happen, often simultaneously;

- Monitoring equipment is attached to the patient;
- IV access is obtained;
- The patient is preoxygenated.

Once all of these have been achieved satisfactorily, the patient is anaesthetized.

Monitoring the patient

This should commence before the induction of anaesthesia and continue until the patient has recovered from the effects of anaesthesia, and the information generated should be recorded in the patient's notes. The type and number of monitors used depend upon a variety of factors including:

- type of operation and operative technique;
- anaesthetic technique used;
- present and previous health of the patient;
- equipment available and the anaesthetist's ability to use it;
- preferences of the anaesthetist;
- any research being undertaken.

The AAGBI recommends certain monitoring devices as *essential* for the safe conduct of anaesthesia. These are: ECG, non-invasive blood pressure, pulse oximeter, capnometry, and vapour concentration analysis. Clearly the latter two are only used after general anaesthesia has commenced. In addition, a peripheral nerve stimulator and temperature monitor should be *immediately available*. Finally, additional equipment *will be required* in certain cases, to monitor, for example, invasive blood pressure, urine output, CVP, and various haemodynamic parameters.

There is good evidence that monitoring reduces the risks of adverse incidents and accidents. The combination of pulse oximetry, capnography, and blood pressure monitoring will detect the majority of serious incidents before there has been serious harm to the patient. Ultimately, monitoring supplements clinical observation; there is no substitute for the presence of a trained and experienced anaesthetist throughout the entire operative procedure.

Monitoring is not without its own potential hazards:

- faulty equipment may endanger the patient, for example from electrocution secondary to faulty earthing;
- the anaesthetist may act on faulty data, instituting inappropriate treatment;
- the patient may be harmed by the complications of the technique to establish invasive monitoring, for example pneumothorax following central venous catheterization.

Ultimately, too many monitors may distract the anaesthetist from recognizing problems occurring in other areas.

Intravenous access

The superficial veins on the back of the hand (*dorsal metacarpal veins*) and forearm (*cephalic and basilic veins*) are most commonly used for IV access. Veins in the antecubital fossa tend to be used either in an emergency situation or when attempts to cannulate more peripheral veins have failed. It must be remembered that the brachial artery, the median nerve, and branches of the medial and lateral cutaneous nerves of the arm are in close proximity to the antecubital veins and easily damaged by needles or extravasated drugs. A cannula must not be sited in a patient's arm on the side where they have undergone clearance of axillary lymph nodes for malignant disease unless there is no alternative, because of the risk of exacerbating lymphoedema. The size of the cannula inserted will depend upon its purpose: large-diameter cannulas are required for giving fluid rapidly, smaller ones are adequate for giving drugs and maintenance fluids. Peripheral venous cannulation is an essential skill, best learnt under the supervision of an anaesthetist, rather that reading about it! Complications of peripheral venous cannulation are shown in Table 3.1.

A small amount of local anaesthetic (0.2 mL of lignocaine 1%) should be infiltrated into the skin at the site chosen for venepuncture using a 25 gauge (0.5 mm) needle, particularly if a large (>18 gauge, 1.2 mm) cannula is used. This reduces pain, and makes the patient less likely to move and less resistant to further attempts.

As with any procedure where there is a risk of contact with body fluids, gloves should be worn by the operator.

Central venous cannulation

This usually takes place after the patient has been anaesthetized to allow monitoring of the

Table 3.1 Complications of peripheral venous cannulation.

- *Failure* Attempt cannulation distally in a limb and work proximally. If multiple attempts are required, fluid or drugs will not leak from previous puncture sites.
- *Haematoma* Usually secondary to the above with inadequate pressure applied over the puncture site to prevent bleeding, and made worse by forgetting to remove the tourniquet!
- *Extravasation of fluid or drugs* Failing to recognize that the cannula is not within the vein before use. May cause damage to the surrounding tissues.
- *Damage to local structures* Secondary to poor technique and lack of knowledge of the local anatomy.
- *Air embolus* Most likely following cannulation of a central vein (see below).
- *Shearing of the cannula* Usually a result of trying to reintroduce the needle after it has been withdrawn. The safest action is to withdraw the whole cannula and re-attempt at another site.
- *Thrombophlebitis* Related to the length of time the vein is in use and irritation caused by the substances flowing through it. High concentrations of drugs and fluids with extremes of pH or high osmolality are the main causes, for example antibiotics, calcium chloride, sodium bicarbonate. Once a vein shows signs of thrombophlebitis (i.e. tender, red, and deteriorating flow) the cannula must be removed to prevent subsequent infection or thrombosis.

cardiovascular system or to give certain drugs (e.g. inotropes). Rarely, it is required before the anaesthetic is given because of lack of or inadequate peripheral venous access (e.g. in a patient who has a history of IV drug abuse). It is included at this point for completeness. There are many different types of equipment and approaches to the central veins, and the following is intended as an outline. It is now recommended that an ultrasound scanner is used to detect central veins and guide the insertion of the needle into the vein (Fig. 3.1).

Central veins can be accessed via the antecubital fossa. This route has now been replaced by use of direct cannulation of one of the central veins, and will not be considered further.

The internal jugular vein

This approach is associated with the highest incidence of success (95%), and a low rate of complications (Table 3.2). The right internal jugular offers certain advantages: there is a 'straight line' to the heart, the apical pleura does not rise as high on this side, and the main thoracic duct is on the left.

Subclavian vein

This can be approached by both the supra- and infraclavicular routes. Both are technically more difficult than the internal jugular route, and there is a significant incidence of causing a pneumothorax (approximately 2%). The main advantages of this route are comfort for the patient and low risk of infection during long-term use.

Bilateral attempts at central venous cannulation must not be made because of the risk of airway obstruction due to haematoma formation in the neck or bilateral pneumothoraces.

Equipment for central venous catheterization

The techniques commonly used for percutaneous cannulation of the central veins are:

- *Catheter over needle*: similar to a peripheral IV cannula, the main difference is that the cannula is longer to ensure that the tip lies in the correct position within a central vein.
- *Seldinger technique*: the vein is punctured initially percutaneously using a small-diameter needle. A flexible guidewire is then passed down the needle into the vein and the needle carefully withdrawn, leaving the wire behind. The catheter is now passed over the wire into the vein, sometimes preceded by a dilator. The advantage of this method is that the initial use of a small needle increases the chance of successful venepuncture and reduces the risk of damage to the vein.

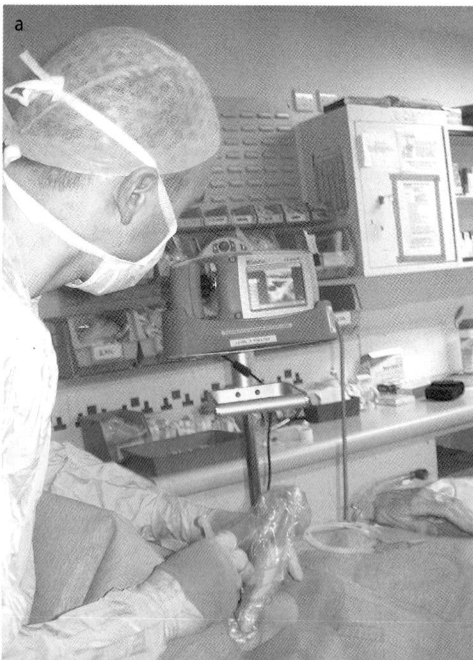

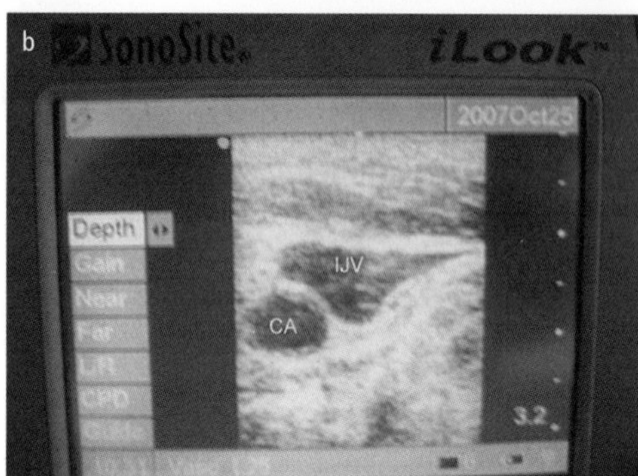

Figure 3.1 (a) Ultrasound guidance being used to insert a CVP catheter, (b) screen view showing the internal jugular vein (IJV) and carotid artery (CA).

> Whenever a central venous catheter is inserted, a chest X-ray must be taken to ensure that the catheter is correctly positioned with the tip at the junction of SVC and right atrium and that a pneumothorax has not been caused.

Table 3.2 Complications of central venous cannulation.

- Arterial puncture and bleeding causing haematoma or haemothorax
- Air embolus
- Venous thrombosis
- Pneumothorax
- Thoracic duct injury (left side) and chylothorax
- Hydrothorax if the catheter is intrapleural and fluid given
- Bacteraemia
- Septicaemia
- Soft tissue infection at puncture site
- Injury to nerves:
  - brachial plexus
  - recurrent laryngeal
  - phrenic

Preoxygenation

At the end of expiration, the lungs contain a significant volume of air that acts as a reservoir (the functional residual capacity, FRC). Amongst other things, this prevents hypoxaemia during brief periods of breath-holding. However, when breathing room air the vast majority of the FRC is nitrogen. The purpose of preoxygenation is to replace the nitrogen with oxygen, thereby significantly increasing the length of time a patient can be apnoeic (or not ventilated) without becoming hypoxic; effectively 'buying time' for the anaesthetist in case of difficulty. Preoxygenation is usually achieved by getting the patient to breathe 100% oxygen via a close-fitting facemask for about 3 min or until the oxygen concentration in expired gas exceeds 85%. In an emergency situation, a reasonable degree of preoxygenation can be achieved by asking a cooperative patient to take four vital capacity breaths of 100% oxygen via an anaesthetic circuit with a tight-sealing facemask.

Induction of anaesthesia

IV drugs are the most frequently used method of inducing anaesthesia. The drug dose is calculated, taking into account the patient's age and any comorbidities, and then given over 20–30 s. This method is generally preferred both by the patient, as consciousness is lost rapidly, and by the anaesthetist because pharyngeal reflexes are depressed, allowing the insertion of an airway device. There are a number of potential disadvantages:

- Patients often become apnoeic. This may necessitate manual ventilation until spontaneous ventilation resumes.
- There will be a varying degree of hypotension. This will depend on the drug, dose used, speed given, and 'fitness' of the patient.
- There may be loss of airway patency. This can usually be overcome by a combination of basic airway opening manoeuvres, insertion of an oropharyngeal airway or use of a LMA.

Inhalational induction of anaesthesia is an alternative. It is achieved by the patient breathing a gradually increasing concentration of an inhalational drug in oxygen or a mixture of oxygen and nitrous oxide. Its advantages are that it can be used in:

- Patients with a lack of suitable veins. Rather than subject the patient to repeated attempts at venepuncture, anaesthesia is induced and, as most drugs are vasodilators, venepuncture is then possible.
- An uncooperative child and patients with a needle phobia. Venous access can be obtained after induction.
- Patients with airway compromise, in which an IV drug may cause apnoea and loss of airway patency. Ventilation and oxygenation become impossible, with catastrophic results. Inhalation induction preserves spontaneous ventilation and, if airway patency is threatened, further uptake of anaesthetic is prevented, limiting the problem.

Potential disadvantages include:

- Unconsciousness occurs more slowly than with an IV drug.
- Most inhalational drugs are unpleasant to breathe. Currently, sevoflurane is the most popular anaesthetic used for this technique.
- Hypotension and a fall in cardiac output occur with increasing concentrations. This may be difficult to treat until IV access is obtained.
- The combination of hypercapnia, as a result of respiratory depression, and the vasodilator effect of these drugs leads to increased cerebral blood flow, making this technique unsuitable in patients with raised ICP.

As the concentration of inhalational increases, there is progressive reduction in the ventilatory activity of the intercostal muscles, muscle tone generally is also reduced, and laryngeal reflexes are lost. The pupils start by becoming dilated, then slightly constricted, and finally gradually dilate. This point is referred to as 'surgical anaesthesia'. Any further increase in depth of anaesthesia will result in diaphragmatic paralysis and cardiovascular collapse.

As well as the above, the anaesthetic will have effects on all of the other body systems, which will need appropriate monitoring.

Maintaining the airway

General anaesthesia frequently causes the patient's airway to become obstructed following loss of tone in the muscles of the tongue and pharynx (Fig. 3.2). The easiest way to restore patency is through basic airway manoeuvres; a combination of the head tilt, chin lift (Fig. 3.3), and jaw thrust (Fig. 3.4), in conjunction with an oro- or nasopharyngeal airway. Although a patent airway can be maintained in the majority of patients in this manner, it is increasingly uncommon as it severely restricts any further activity by the anaesthetist. This problem has been overcome by the use of the LMA. The best method of providing and securing a clear airway in patients is tracheal intubation, but this is not appropriate in all patients.

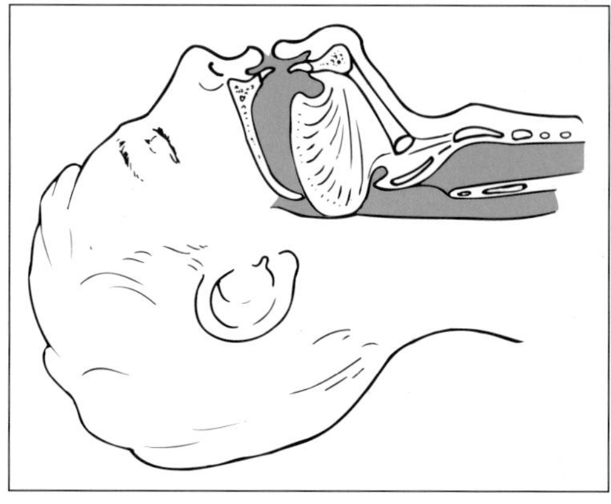

Figure 3.2 Sagittal section of the head and neck showing how the tongue contributes to airway obstruction.

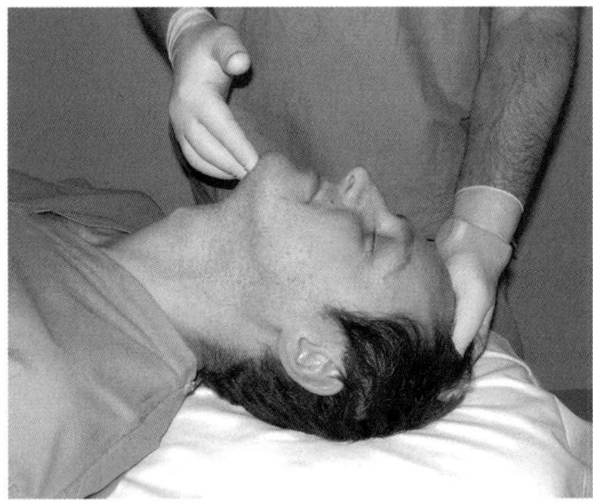

Figure 3.3 Head tilt, chin lift.

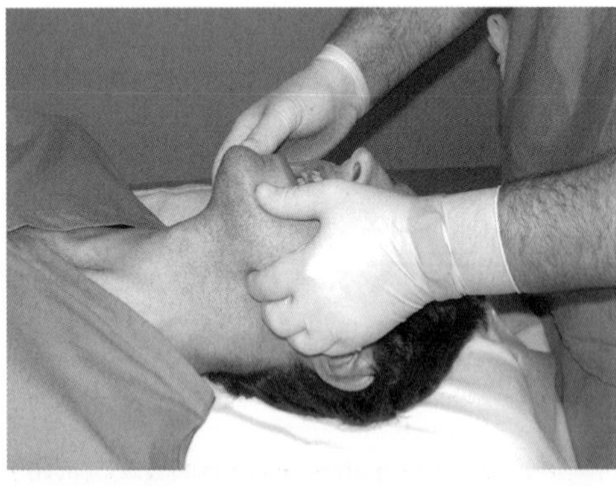

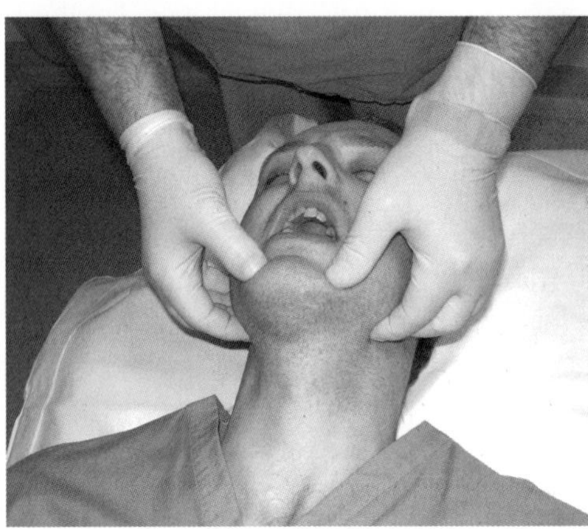

Figure 3.4 Jaw thrust. The application of pressure is behind the angles of the mandible. The thumbs can be used to open the mouth.

Oropharyngeal airway

Estimate the size required by comparing the airway length with the vertical distance between the patient's incisor teeth (or, if edentulous, the corner of the mouth) and the angle of the jaw. Then insert the airway initially 'upside down', as far as the back of the hard palate, before rotating it 180° and fully inserting until the flange lies in front of the teeth (or gums in an edentulous patient) (Fig. 3.5a–d).

Nasopharyngeal airway

Chose an appropriately sized airway, 7 mm for women, 8 mm for men, check the patency of the nostril to be used (usually the right), and lubricate the airway. The airway is then inserted along the floor of the nose, with the bevel facing medially to avoid catching the turbinates (Fig. 3.6a–c). A safety pin may be inserted through the flange to prevent inhalation of the airway. If obstruction is encountered, do not use force as severe bleeding may be provoked. Instead, try the other nostril.

Problems with airways

- Although the techniques described so far will create and maintain a patent airway, they offer no protection against aspiration of regurgitated gastric contents.
- Failure to maintain a patent airway: snoring, indrawing of the supraclavicular, suprasternal and intercostal spaces, use of the accessory muscles, or paradoxical respiratory movement (see-saw respiration) suggest obstruction.
- Inability to maintain a good seal between the patient's face and the mask, particularly in those without teeth.
- Fatigue, when holding the mask for prolonged periods.
- The anaesthetist not being free to deal with any other problems that may arise.

The LMA (or similar device) or tracheal intubation may be used to overcome these problems.

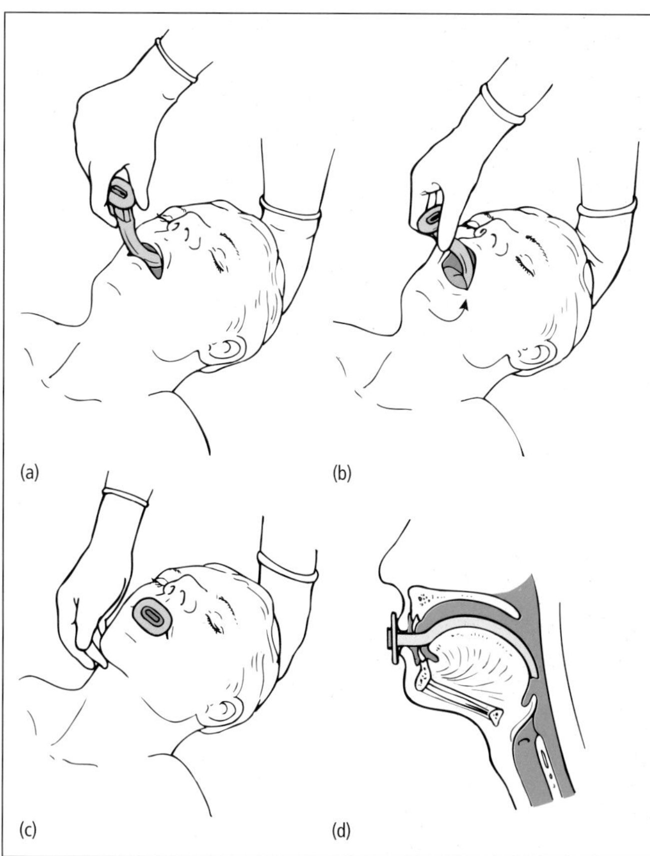

Figure 3.5 (a–d) The sequence for inserting an oropharyngeal airway.

Facemasks

To ensure that the anaesthetic gas mixture is delivered to the patient, a facemask is used. Leakage of gases is minimized by using one that provides a good seal. When holding a facemask in position with the index finger and thumb, the jaw thrust is achieved by lifting the angle of the mandible with the remaining fingers of one or both hands. The overall desired effect is that the patient's mandible is 'lifted' into the mask, rather than the mask being pushed into the face (Fig. 3.7). The patient can now breathe spontaneously or be ventilated.

The LMA

This device is widely used in spontaneously breathing patients as it overcomes some of the problems associated with the techniques described above:

- They are not affected by the shape of the patient's face or the absence of teeth.
- The anaesthetist is not required to hold it in position or maintain a jaw thrust or chin lift, thereby avoiding fatigue and allowing any other problems to be dealt with.
- They *significantly reduce* the risk of aspiration of regurgitated gastric contents, but do not eliminate it completely.
- Their use is *relatively contraindicated* where there is an increased risk of regurgitation, for example in emergency cases, pregnancy, and patients with a hiatus hernia.

In addition to the above, the LMA has proved to be a valuable aid in those patients who are difficult to intubate, as it can usually be inserted to facilitate

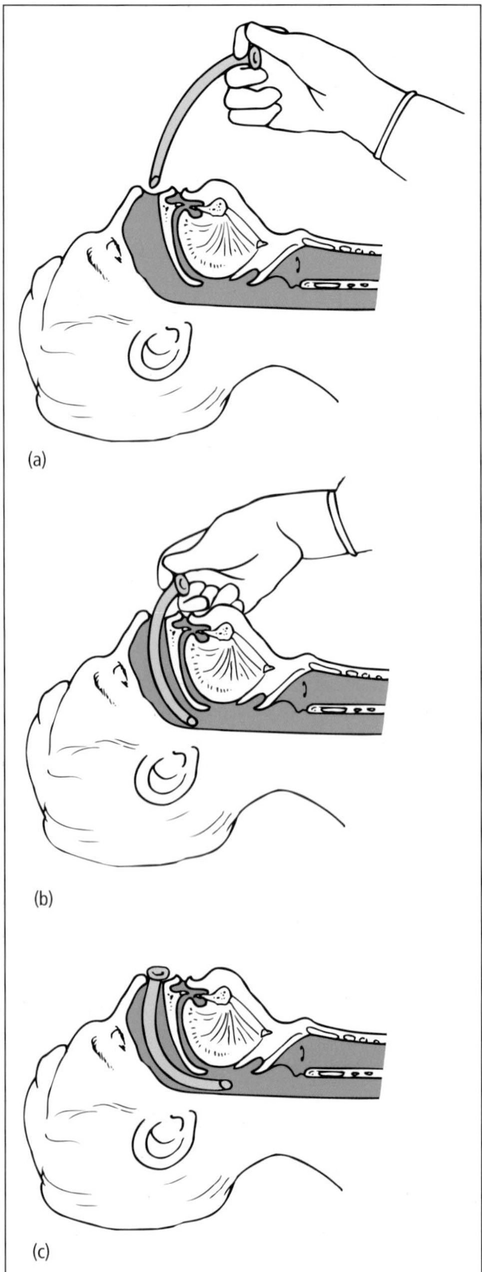

Figure 3.6 (a–c) The sequence for inserting a nasopharyngeal airway.

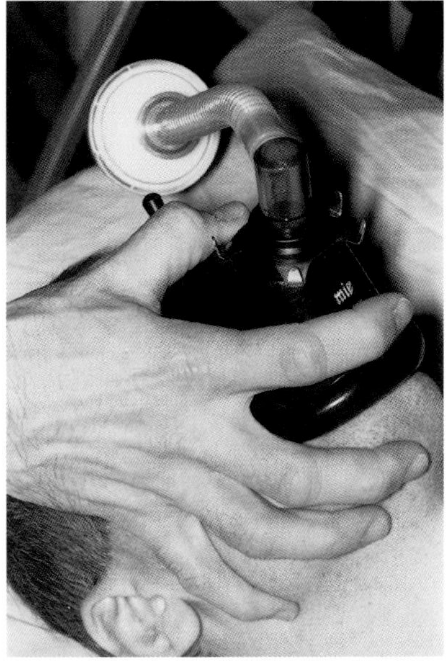

Figure 3.7 Mask being held on a patient's face. View from the side to show use of jaw thrust.

oxygenation while additional help or equipment is obtained (see below).

Insertion of a standard LMA (Fig 3.8a–e)

The patient's reflexes must be suppressed to a level similar to that required for the insertion of an oropharyngeal airway to prevent coughing or laryngospasm.

- The cuff is deflated (Fig. 3.8a) and the mask lightly lubricated.
- A head tilt is performed, the patient's mouth opened fully, and the tip of the mask inserted along the hard palate with the open side facing but not touching the tongue (Fig. 3.8b).
- The mask is further inserted, using the index finger to provide support for the tube (Fig. 3.8c). Eventually, resistance will be felt at the point where the tip of the mask lies at the upper oesophageal sphincter (Fig. 3.8d).
- The cuff is now fully inflated using an air-filled syringe attached to the valve at the end of the pilot tube (Fig. 3.8e).

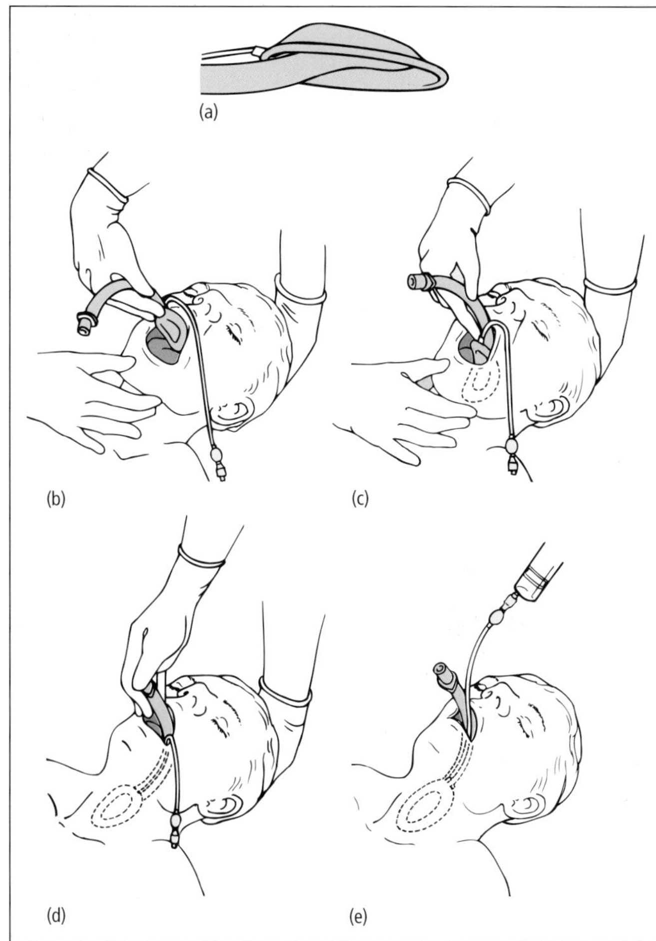

Figure 3.8 (a–e) Sequence for the insertion of a laryngeal mask airway (LMA).

- The laryngeal mask is secured by either a length of bandage or adhesive strapping attached to the protruding tube.
- A 'bite block' may be inserted to reduce the risk of damage to the LMA at recovery.

Tracheal intubation

This requires abolition of the laryngeal reflexes. During anaesthesia, this is achieved by giving a neuromuscular blocking drug. Alternatively, deep inhalational anaesthesia or local anaesthesia of the larynx can be used, but these are generally reserved for patients in whom difficulty with intubation is anticipated, for example in the presence of airway tumours or immobility of the cervical spine. The common indications for tracheal intubation are shown in Table 3.3

Equipment for tracheal intubation

The equipment used will be determined by the circumstances and by the preferences of the individual anaesthetist. The following is a list of the basic needs for *adult oral* intubation.

- *Laryngoscope*: with a curved (Macintosh) blade and functioning light.
- *Tracheal tubes (cuffed)*: in a variety of sizes. The internal diameter is expressed in millimetres and the length in centimetres. They may be lightly lubricated.
  - For males: 8.0–9.0 mm internal diameter, 22–24 cm length.

Table 3.3 Common indications for tracheal intubation.

• Where muscle relaxants are used to facilitate surgery (e.g. abdominal and thoracic surgery), thereby necessitating the use of mechanical ventilation.
• In patients with a full stomach, to protect against aspiration.
• Where the position of the patient would make airway maintenance difficult, for example the lateral or prone position.
• Where there is competition between surgeon and anaesthetist for the airway (e.g. operations on the head and neck).
• Where controlled ventilation is utilized to improve surgical access (e.g. neurosurgery).
• In those patients in whom the airway cannot be satisfactorily maintained by any other technique.
• During cardiopulmonary resuscitation.

  - For females: 7.0–8.0 mm internal diameter, 20–22 cm length.
- *Syringe*: to inflate the cuff once the tube is in place.
- *Catheter mount*: or 'elbow' to connect the tube to the anaesthetic system or ventilator tubing.
- *Suction*: switched on and immediately to hand in case the patient vomits or regurgitates.
- *Capnometer*: a device to detect carbon dioxide in expired gas (see below) thereby confirming placement of the tube in the airway.
- *Stethoscope*: to check ventilation of both lungs is occurring by listening for breath sounds during ventilation.
- *Extras*: a semi-rigid introducer to help mould the tube to a particular shape; Magill's forceps, designed to reach into the pharynx to remove debris or direct the tip of a tube; different size or style laryngoscope blades (e.g. McCoy); bandage or tape to secure the tube.

The technique of oral intubation

Following IV induction, it is good practice to ensure that the patient can be ventilated via a facemask before giving the neuromuscular blocking drug to facilitate intubation. If intubation then proves to be unexpectedly difficult or impossible, the anaesthetist knows that oxygenation can be maintained and the patient will come to no harm. Along with the neuromuscular blocking drug, an IV opioid is often given to reduce the cardiovascular response to intubation. During the time it takes for a non-depolarizing neuromuscular blocker to reach maximal effect, there will be a period of apnoea. The patient will need to be ventilated manually with a mixture of oxygen and an inhalational drug to maintain anaesthesia. Once the degree of neuromuscular block is adequate, direct laryngoscopy is performed.

With the patient's head on a small pillow, the neck is flexed and the head extended at the atlanto-occipital joint, the 'sniffing the morning air' position. The patient's mouth is fully opened using the index finger and thumb of the *right* hand in a scissor action. The laryngoscope is held in the *left* hand and the blade introduced into the mouth along the right-hand side of the tongue, displacing it to the left. The blade is advanced until the tip lies in the gap between the base of the tongue and the epiglottis, the vallecula. Force is then applied *in the direction in which the handle of the laryngoscope is pointing*. The effort comes from the upper arm not the wrist, to lift the tongue and epiglottis. This exposes the larynx, seen as a triangular opening, with the apex anteriorly and the whitish coloured true cords laterally (Fig. 3.9).

The tracheal tube is introduced into the right side of the mouth, advanced and *seen to pass through the cords* until the cuff lies just below them. The tube is then held firmly, the laryngoscope is carefully removed, and the cuff is inflated sufficiently to prevent any leak during ventilation. The patient is now ventilated manually while the position of the tube is confirmed, and it is secured to the patient using adhesive tape or cotton tape.

For some types of surgery, for example oral surgery, nasotracheal intubation is used so that the tube is out of the surgical field. A well-lubricated tube is introduced, usually via the right nostril,

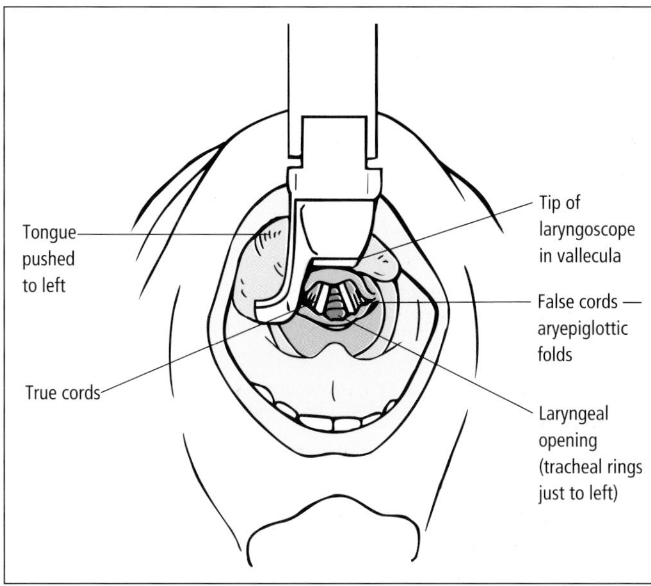

Figure 3.9 A view of the larynx at laryngoscopy.

along the floor of the nose with the bevel pointing medially to avoid damage to the turbinates. It is advanced into the oropharynx, where it is usually visualized using a laryngoscope in the manner described above. It can then either be advanced directly into the larynx by pushing on the proximal end, or the tip picked up with Magill's forceps (which are designed not to impair the view of the larynx) and directed into the larynx. The procedure then continues as for oral intubation.

Confirming the position of the tracheal tube

Every tracheal tube inserted ***must*** have its position checked. This can be achieved using a number of techniques of varying reliability:

- *Measuring the CO_2 in expired gas (capnometry)*: the presence of CO_2 in expired gas indicates that the tube is in the airway; less than 0.2% indicates oesophageal intubation. However, it does not indicate when the tube has been inserted too far and lies in a main bronchus. This can usually be determined by listening to both sides of the chest for equality of breath sounds.
- *Oesophageal detector*: a 50 mL syringe is attached to the tracheal tube and the plunger rapidly withdrawn. If the tracheal tube is in the oesophagus, resistance is felt and air cannot be aspirated; if it is in the trachea, air is easily aspirated.
- *Direct visualization*: of the tracheal tube passing between the vocal cords.
- *Fogging*: on clear plastic tube connectors during expiration.
- Less reliable signs are:
  - diminished breath sounds on auscultation;
  - decreased chest movement on ventilation;
  - gurgling sounds over the epigastrium and 'burping' sounds as gas escapes;
  - a decrease in oxygen saturation detected by pulse oximetry. This occurs late, particularly if the patient has been preoxygenated.

Complications of tracheal intubation

The following complications are the more common ones, not an attempt to cover all eventualities.

Hypoxia

Due to:

- *Unrecognized oesophageal intubation.* If there is any doubt about the position of the tube it should be removed and the patient ventilated via a facemask. This is most likely to occur when capnometry is unavailable.

• *Failed intubation and inability to ventilate the patient.* This is a rare event and usually a result of abnormal anatomy or airway pathology. In elective patients, it may be predictable at the preoperative assessment (see Chapter 1).

• *Failed ventilation after intubation.* Possible causes include the tube becoming kinked, blocked, or disconnected, severe bronchospasm, and tension pneumothorax. It may also be due to failure of the anaesthetic gas supply.

• *Aspiration.* Regurgitated gastric contents can cause blockage of the airways directly, or secondary to laryngeal spasm and bronchospasm. Cricoid pressure can be used to reduce the risk of regurgitation prior to intubation (see below).

Trauma

• *Direct.* During laryngoscopy and insertion of the endotracheal tube, damage to lips, teeth, tongue, pharynx, larynx, trachea, and nose and nasopharynx during nasal intubation; causing soft tissue swelling or bleeding.

• *Indirect.* To the recurrent laryngeal nerves, and the cervical spine and cord, particularly where there is pre-existing degenerative disease or trauma.

Reflex activity

• *Hypertension and arrhythmias.* Occurs in response to laryngoscopy and intubation, and may jeopardize patients with coronary artery disease. In patients at risk, specific action is taken to attenuate the response, for example pretreatment with beta-blockers or potent analgesics (fentanyl, remifentanil).

• *Vomiting.* This may be stimulated when laryngoscopy is attempted in patients who are inadequately anaesthetized. It is more frequent when there is material in the stomach, for example in emergencies when the patient is not starved, in patients with intestinal obstruction, or when gastric emptying is delayed, as after opiate analgesics or following trauma.

• *Laryngeal spasm.* Reflex adduction of the vocal cords as a result of stimulation of the epiglottis or larynx.

Difficult intubation

Occasionally it is not possible to visualize the larynx, which makes it difficult to intubate the trachea. This may have been predicted at the preoperative assessment or may be unexpected. A variety of techniques have been described to help solve this problem and include the following:

• Manipulation of the thyroid cartilage (BURP manoeuvre) using **b**ackward, **u**pward, **r**ightward **p**ressure (patient's right) by an assistant to try and bring the larynx or its posterior aspect into view.

• At laryngoscopy, a 60 cm long gum elastic bougie is inserted blindly into the trachea, over which the tracheal tube is 'railroaded' into place.

• A fibreoptic bronchoscope is introduced into the trachea via the mouth or nose, and is used as a guide over which a tube can be passed into the trachea. This technique has the advantage that it can be used in either anaesthetized or awake patients.

• An LMA or ILM can be inserted and used as a conduit to pass a tracheal tube directly or via a fibreoptic bronchoscope.

Failed intubation

Despite utilizing the techniques described above, the patient cannot be intubated. The incidence of failed intubation will depend on a number of factors, including the skill and experience of the anaesthetist and the type of cases being undertaken. The following plans concentrate on *unexpected failed intubation where oxygenation can be maintained.* The immediate management in these circumstances will depend upon:

• type of neuromuscular blocker used, either depolarizing or non-depolarizing;

• urgency of surgery (and the likelihood of a full stomach);

• need for intubation.

Anaesthesia for elective surgery

Assume that the patient is starved, minimizing the risk of aspiration, and a non-depolarizing neuromuscular blocker given to facilitate tracheal intubation.

- Get help.
- Administer 100% oxygen via a facemask.
- Ventilate gently to minimize the risk of gastric distension, try one- or two-person technique, use an oral and/or nasal airway.

Oxygenation and ventilation successful

Maintain anaesthesia with inhalational agent in oxygen.

Intubation essential for surgery:

- Attempt fibreoptic intubation.
- Attempt intubation using an LMA or ILM.
- Maintain anaesthesia and ventilation using an LMA or facemask until neuromuscular block can be reversed; awaken patient and plan for elective fibreoptic intubation.

Intubation not essential for surgery:

- Use an LMA, Pro-seal® LMA or Combitube®.
- Consider using a regional anaesthetic technique.

Anaesthesia for emergency surgery

Assuming the patient has a full stomach, a rapid-sequence induction (RSI) technique of preoxygenation, cricoid pressure, and suxamethonium has been used to facilitate intubation (see page 80):

- Get help.
- Maintain cricoid pressure.
- Give 100% oxygen via facemask.
- Maximize head tilt and jaw thrust.
- Use an oral and/or nasal airway.
- Ventilate gently to minimize the risk of gastric distension, try one- or two-person technique.
- Consider reducing cricoid pressure if ventilation difficult.

Oxygenation and ventilation successful

Surgery essential:

- Continue anaesthesia with inhalational agent in oxygen.
- Maintain airway with LMA, Pro-seal® LMA or Combitube®.

Surgery not essential:

- Maintain oxygenation and allow patient to recover.
- Plan alternative technique.

Intubation essential for surgery. Depending on skills available:

- Insert LMA or ILM and use as a conduit for fibreoptic intubation; or
- allow the patient to recover, empty the stomach via a nasogastric tube, and use awake fibreoptic intubation under local anaesthesia.

Intubation not essential for surgery:

- Use a LMA, Pro-seal® LMA or Combitube®.
- Consider allowing the patient to wake up, and use a regional anaesthetic technique.

Failed intubation, failed ventilation

Although failure of intubation may occur relatively frequently, the combination of failed intubation and failed mask ventilation (often referred to as 'can't intubate, can't ventilate') is very rare and estimated to occur in fewer than 1 : 10 000 cases. Whatever the surgical urgency, if intubation fails and the patient cannot be oxygenated via a facemask, LMA, or any other means, they are in immediate danger of dying:

- GET HELP.
- Give 100% oxygen via facemask, use the emergency oxygen flush.
- Maximum head tilt, and jaw thrust.
- Use oral and/or nasal airway.
- Try LMA, Proseal® LMA, ILM, Combitube®, whichever most familiar with.
- Perform needle cricothyroidotomy and start oxygen insufflation.
- In any situation other than surgery for an immediately life-threatening condition, maintain oxygenation and unconsciousness (using TIVA) until neuromuscular block has worn off or is reversible.
- In life-threatening circumstances, maintain oxygenation, and secure the airway using an alternative technique (tracheostomy, fibreoptic intubation).

Any patient whose airway has been traumatized, either as a result of repeated attempts at intubation or following surgical intervention, is at risk of developing oedema and airway obstruction at extubation. These patients should be admitted to an appropriate critical care area postoperatively and may require endoscopy prior to extubation.

Full details of the difficulties encountered and any solutions must be documented in the patient's notes. The patient must be given verbal and written details (consider a 'Medic Alert'-type device) and details sent to his or her GP.

Needle cricothyroidotomy

This technique is used only ***when all others have failed to maintain oxygenation***. The cricothyroid membrane is identified and punctured using a large-bore cannula (12–14 gauge) attached to a syringe. Aspiration of air confirms that the tip of the cannula lies within the trachea. The cannula is then angled to about 45° caudally and advanced off the needle into the trachea (Fig. 3.10a). In order to overcome the high resistance of the narrow cannula lumen, the oxygen delivered must be from a high-pressure supply (Fig. 3.10b). While holding the cannula in place, oxygen is insufflated for 1 s, followed by a 4 s rest. Expiration occurs via the upper airway as normal, along with the escape of excess gas during insufflation. This technique adequately oxygenates the patient but only results in minimal CO_2 elimination, and is therefore limited to about 30 min use while help is obtained and a definitive airway is created. Extreme care must be taken if this technique is used in the presence of upper airway obstruction. Progressively more oxygen is delivered to the lungs by the high-pressure source that cannot escape, eventually causing a pneumothorax.

Maintenance of anaesthesia

The effects of the IV drug used for induction of anaesthesia wear off after a few minutes and unconsciousness must be maintained in some other way. This can be achieved using one of a variety of inhalational anaesthetics in oxygen with or without nitrous oxide, or by an IV infusion of a drug (TIVA), most commonly propofol. Whether the patient breathes spontaneously or is ventilated, the principles are similar.

Inhalational anaesthesia

The patient must receive:

- A sufficient concentration of oxygen to prevent hypoxia.
- A sufficient concentration of anaesthetic drug to ensure unconsciousness.
- A sufficient flow of fresh gases to prevent hypercarbia.

In order to achieve these, the composition of the gas mixture is carefully monitored. The inspired oxygen concentration is usually maintained between 30 and 50%. This will be lower than the concentration being delivered by the anaesthetic machine when a circle system is being used because of the dilutional effect of the expired gases. The anaesthetic drug used is maintained at an appropriate end-tidal concentration depending upon the patient, the surgical stimulus, and the concurrent use of analgesic drugs.

In the spontaneously breathing patient, inadequate anaesthesia for the intensity of the surgical stimulus, for example when surgery starts, will result in an increased respiratory rate and the patient may move as a result of reflex activity. In addition there may be an increase in heart rate and blood pressure. As a result the anaesthetist will increase the concentration of anaesthetic drug accordingly to deepen the level of unconsciousness. It may also be appropriate to halt surgery temporarily while this is achieved.

In the patient who has been given neuromuscular blocking drugs and is being ventilated, the anaesthetist must anticipate the need for changes in the depth of anaesthesia as the patient's ventilation will not change and they cannot move. Furthermore, if potent opioid analgesics have been given, changes in cardiovascular signs may be minimal. Consequently there is the possibility that the depth of anaesthesia is inadequate and the patient may be aware and unable to communicate this.

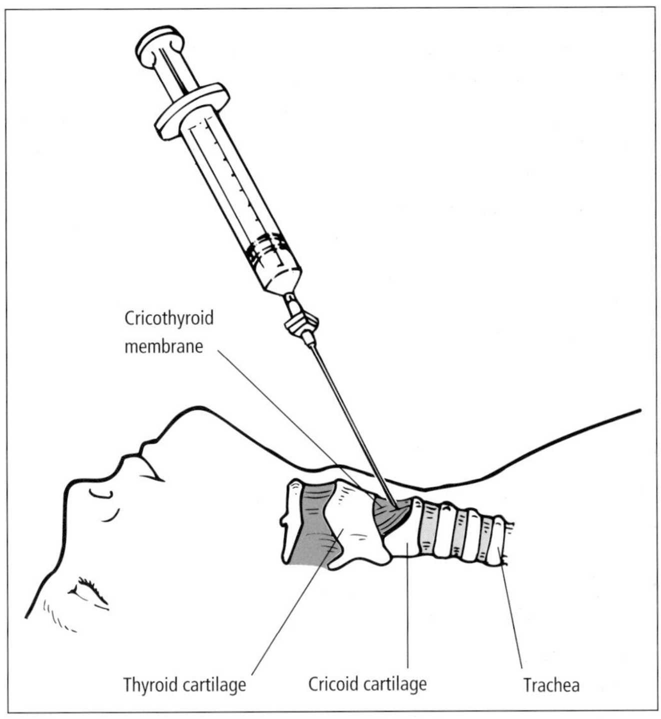

(a)

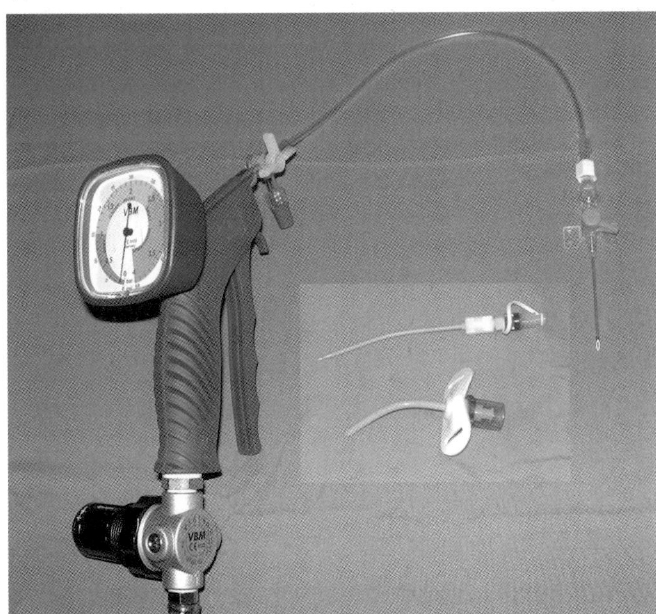

(b)

Figure 3.10 (a) Needle cricothyroidotomy, (b) oxygen delivery system (Manujet) attached to an IV cannula. The pressure of oxygen delivered is controlled by the lower black knob and displayed on the dial. Inset: purpose-made cannula and stylet for cricothyroid puncture.

TIVA using propofol

With this technique, an appropriate brain concentration of propofol must be achieved and maintained to prevent awareness and any response to surgery. The simplest way is to give the usual IV induction dose, followed by repeated injections at intervals depending on the patient's response. This method can be used for short procedures, but for maintenance over a longer period it is more common to use a microprocessor-controlled infusion pump. This is more accurate and reliable as it uses the patient's weight and age to calculate the rate of infusion required to achieve a constant plasma (and brain) concentration. Having entered the appropriate data and started the pump, an initial rapid infusion is given to render the patient unconscious, followed by an infusion at a slower rate to maintain anaesthesia. This is often referred to as 'target-controlled infusion' (TCI). The infusion rate, and hence plasma concentration, can also be adjusted manually, to take account of individual patient variation and the degree of surgical stimulation, in the same way that the concentration of a inhalational anaesthetic from the vaporizer can be changed.

Propofol alone can be used to maintain anaesthesia, but the infusion rates required are very high, with significant cardiovascular side-effects. It is usually combined with IV opioids, given either as repeated injections (e.g. fentanyl) or as an infusion (e.g. remifentanil). An alternative is to use a regional anaesthetic technique for analgesia. If muscle relaxation is required, neuromuscular blocking drugs are given and the patient is usually ventilated with oxygen-enriched air. Nitrous oxide can be used, but this is not strictly TIVA and some of the advantages are lost.

Advantages of total intravenous anaesthesia

- The potential toxic effects of the inhalational anaesthetics are avoided.
- The problems associated with nitrous oxide can be avoided.
- A better quality of recovery is claimed.
- It may be beneficial in certain types of surgery, for example neurosurgery.
- Pollution is reduced.

Disadvantages of total intravenous anaesthesia

- Secure, reliable IV access is required.
- Risk of awareness if IV infusion fails.
- Cost of electronic infusion pumps.
- May cause profound hypotension.

Spontaneous ventilation

Theoretically any operation can be done with the patient breathing spontaneously. However, body cavity surgery, for example laparotomy, requires the inhibition of autonomic reflexes and significant muscle relaxation. This can only be achieved with relatively high concentrations of an inhaled or IV drug that result in respiratory depression or even apnoea. Furthermore, at the end of surgery, as high concentrations of drugs have been given, it will take longer to excrete or eliminate them, thereby prolonging the patient's recovery. Consequently, spontaneous ventilation is used predominantly for peripheral or body surface surgery, where minimal muscle relaxation is required and autonomic reflexes can be modified by the careful titration of small doses of IV opioids or the use of regional anaesthetic techniques.

Mechanical ventilation

The indications for using mechanical ventilation will vary amongst anaesthetists, but most would agree with using it in the following situations:

- Where neuromuscular blocking drugs are used to facilitate surgical access, for example laparotomy.
- During thoracotomy to prevent paradoxical movement.
- When the anaesthetic technique will result in an unacceptable degree of respiratory depression.
- To allow control of carbon dioxide and cerebral blood flow during neurosurgery.

Increasingly, patients are ventilated during long surgical procedures and when they have been intubated.

The anaesthetist will have to ensure that the correct ventilator settings are used for each patient to ensure adequate alveolar ventilation while minimizing the adverse effects of positive pressure. This will require setting of:

- Tidal volume and respiratory rate or, minute volume and tidal volume. This will then determine respiratory rate.
- The mode of ventilation (volume or pressure controlled).
- The inspiratory and expiratory times.
- Peak inspiratory pressure.
- The use of positive end expiratory pressure (PEEP) if required.

Modern ventilators have a range of integral monitors and alarms that can be set to indicate if the desired ventilation is not being achieved.

The effects of positive pressure ventilation

The reversal of the normal inspiratory pressure changes seen during mechanical ventilation has a number of important effects:

- There is an increase in the physiological dead space relative to the tidal volume and in ventilation/perfusion (V/Q) mismatch, both acting to impair oxygenation. An inspired oxygen concentration of at least 30% is used to compensate for this and prevent hypoxaemia.
- The arterial partial pressure of carbon dioxide ($PaCO_2$) is dependent on alveolar ventilation. Hyperventilation results in hypocapnia, causing a respiratory alkalosis. This 'shifts' the oxyhaemoglobin dissociation curve to the left, increasing the affinity of haemoglobin for oxygen. Hypocapnia will induce vasoconstriction in many organs, including the brain and heart, reducing blood flow. Underventilation will lead to hypercapnia, causing a respiratory acidosis. The effects on the oxyhaemoglobin dissociation curve are the opposite of those above, along with stimulation of the sympathetic nervous system causing vasodilatation, hypertension, tachycardia, and arrhythmias.
- Excessive tidal volume may cause overdistension of the alveoli. In patients with pre-existing lung disease, this may cause a pneumothorax, and, if it continues long term, a condition called ventilator-induced lung injury.
- The positive intrathoracic pressure reduces venous return to the heart and cardiac output.
- Both systemic and pulmonary blood flow are reduced, the latter further increasing V/Q mismatch.

Local and regional anaesthesia

When referring to local and regional techniques and the drugs used, the terms 'analgesia' and 'anaesthesia' are used loosely and interchangeably. For clarity and consistency, the following terms will be used:

- *Analgesia.* The state when only relief of pain is provided. This may allow some minor surgical procedures to be performed, for example infiltration analgesia for suturing.
- *Anaesthesia.* The state when analgesia is accompanied by muscle relaxation, usually to allow major surgery to be undertaken. Regional anaesthesia may be used alone or in combination with general anaesthesia.

The role of local and regional anaesthesia

Regional anaesthesia is not just an answer to the problem of anaesthesia in patients regarded as not well enough for general anaesthesia. The decision to use any of these techniques should be based on the advantages offered to both the patient and the surgeon. The following are some of the considerations taken into account:

- Analgesia or anaesthesia is provided predominantly in the area required, thereby avoiding the systemic effects of drugs.
- In patients with chronic respiratory disease, spontaneous ventilation can be preserved and respiratory depressant drugs avoided.
- There is generally less disturbance of the control of coexisting systemic disease requiring medical therapy, for example diabetes mellitus.
- The airway reflexes are preserved and, in a patient with a full stomach, particularly due to

delayed gastric emptying (e.g. pregnancy), the risk of aspiration is reduced.

• Central neural blockade may improve access and facilitate surgery, for example by causing contraction of the bowel or by providing profound muscle relaxation.

• Blood loss can be reduced with controlled hypotension.

• There is a considerable reduction in the equipment required and the cost of anaesthesia. This may be important in underdeveloped areas.

• When used in conjunction with general anaesthesia, only sufficient anaesthetic (inhalational or IV) is required to maintain unconsciousness, with analgesia and muscle relaxation provided by the regional technique.

• Some techniques can be continued postoperatively to provide pain relief, for example an epidural.

• Complications after major surgery, particularly orthopaedic surgery, are significantly reduced.

> A patient should never be forced to accept a local or regional technique. Initial objections and fears are best alleviated, and usually overcome, by explanation of the advantages and reassurance.

Whenever a local or regional anaesthetic technique is used, facilities for resuscitation must always be immediately available in order that allergic reactions and toxicity can be dealt with effectively. As a minimum, this will include the following:

• Equipment to maintain and secure the airway, give oxygen, and provide ventilation.

• IV cannulae and a range of fluids.

• Drugs, including adrenaline, atropine, vasopressors, and anticonvulsants.

• Suction.

• A surface for the patient that is capable of being tipped head-down.

Local and regional anaesthetic techniques

Local anaesthetics can be used:

• topically to a mucous membrane, for example the eye or urethra;

• for subcutaneous infiltration;

• IV after the application of a tourniquet (intravenous regional anaesthesia (IVRA));

• directly around nerves, for example the brachial plexus;

• in the extradural space ('epidural anaesthesia');

• in the subarachnoid space ('spinal anaesthesia').

The latter two techniques are more correctly called 'central neural blockade'; however, the term 'spinal anaesthesia' is commonly used when local anaesthetic is injected into the subarachnoid space and it is in this context that it will be used. The following is a brief introduction to some of the more popular regional anaesthetic techniques; those who require more detail should consult the texts in 'Further reading'.

Infiltration analgesia (Fig. 3.11)

Lignocaine 0.5% is used for short procedures, for example suturing a wound, and 0.5% bupivacaine or chirocaine for pain relief from a surgical incision. A solution containing adrenaline can be used if a large dose or a prolonged effect is required, providing that tissues around end arteries are avoided. Infiltration analgesia is not instantaneous, and lack of patience is the most common reason for failure. The technique used is as follows:

• Calculate the maximum volume of drug that can be used (see page 47).

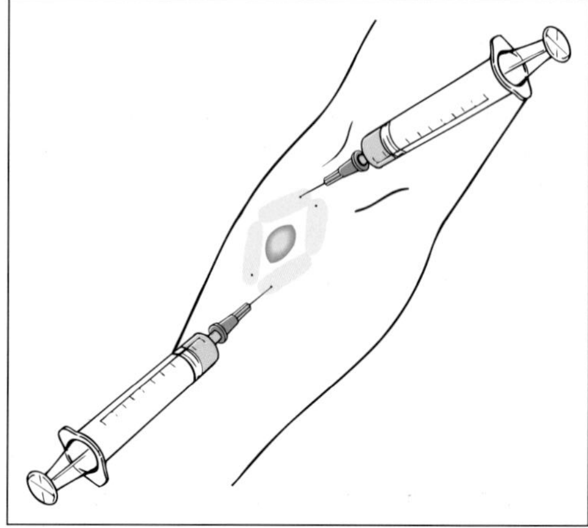

Figure 3.11 Infiltration with local anaesthetic.

- Clean the skin surrounding the wound with an appropriate solution and allow it to dry.
- Insert the needle subcutaneously, avoiding any obvious blood vessels.
- Aspirate to ensure that the tip of the needle does not lie in a blood vessel. If blood is aspirated, discard the syringe and start again.
- Inject the local anaesthetic in a constant flow as the needle is withdrawn. Too rapid injection will cause pain.
- Second and subsequent punctures should be made through an area of skin already anaesthetized.

In a clean wound, local anaesthetic can be injected directly into the exposed wound edge. This technique can also be used at the end of surgery to help reduce wound pain postoperatively.

Brachial plexus block

The nerves of the brachial plexus can be anaesthetized by injecting the local anaesthetic drug either above the level of the clavicle (supraclavicular approach) or where they enter the arm through the axilla along with the axillary artery and vein (axillary approach). A nerve stimulator is used to locate the nerves, and increasingly ultrasound is being used as well to allow more precise insertion of the needle and avoid nerve injury and intravascular injection of the local anaesthetic drug. All of the drugs in Table 2.14 can be used. These techniques can be used for a wide range of surgical procedures below the elbow and will frequently provide good analgesia in the immediate postoperative period. The block may last several hours, and so it is important to warn both the surgeon and patient of this.

Epidural anaesthesia

Epidural (extradural) anaesthesia involves the deposition of a local anaesthetic drug into the potential space *outside* the dura (Fig. 3.12a). This space extends from the craniocervical junction at C1 to the sacrococcygeal membrane, and anaesthesia can theoretically be safely instituted at any level in between. In practice, an epidural is sited adjacent to the nerve roots that supply the surgical site, i.e. the lumbar region is used for pelvic and lower limb surgery and the thoracic region for abdominal surgery. A single injection of local anaesthetic can be given, but more commonly a catheter is inserted into the epidural space and either repeated injections or a constant infusion of a local anaesthetic drug is used.

To aid identification of the epidural space, a technique termed 'loss of resistance' is used. The (Tuohy) needle is advanced until its tip is embedded within the ligamentum flavum (yellow ligament). This blocks the tip and causes marked resistance to attempted injection of either air or saline from a syringe attached to the needle. As the needle is advanced further, the ligament is pierced, resistance disappears dramatically, and air or saline is injected easily. The needle has markings every 1 cm to enable determination of the depth of the epidural space.

A plastic catheter is then inserted into the epidural space via the needle. The catheter is marked at 5 cm intervals to 20 cm, with extra markings every 1 cm between 5 and 15 cm. Knowing how far the catheter has been inserted, as well as the depth of the epidural space, allows calculation of the length of the catheter in the epidural space.

Varying concentrations of local anaesthetics are used depending on what effect is required. For example, bupivacaine or chirocaine 0.5% will be needed for surgical anaesthesia with muscle relaxation, but only 0.1–0.2% for postoperative analgesia. Local anaesthetic will spread from the level of injection both up and down the epidural space. The extent of anaesthesia is determined by:

- The spinal level of insertion of the epidural. For a given volume, spread is greater in the thoracic region than in the lumbar region.
- The volume of local anaesthetic injected.
- Gravity: tipping the patient head-down encourages spread cranially, while head-up tends to limit spread.

The spread of anaesthesia is described with reference to the limits of the dermatomes affected, for example the inguinal ligament, T12; the umbilicus, T10; and the nipples, T4. An opioid is often given with the local anaesthetic to improve the

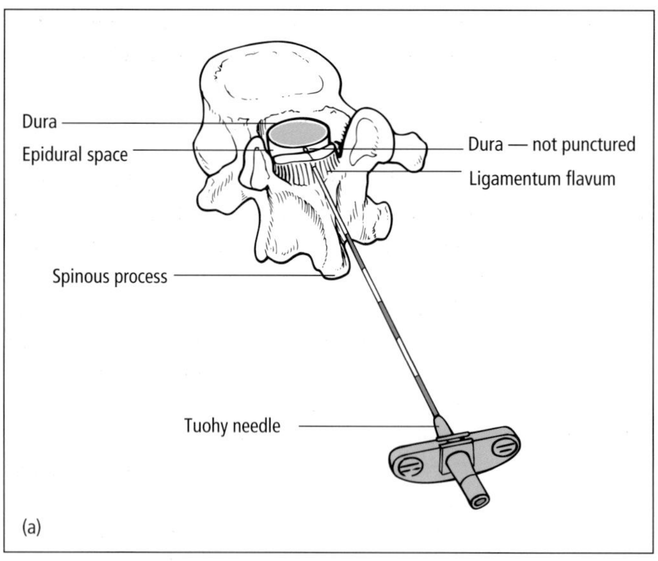

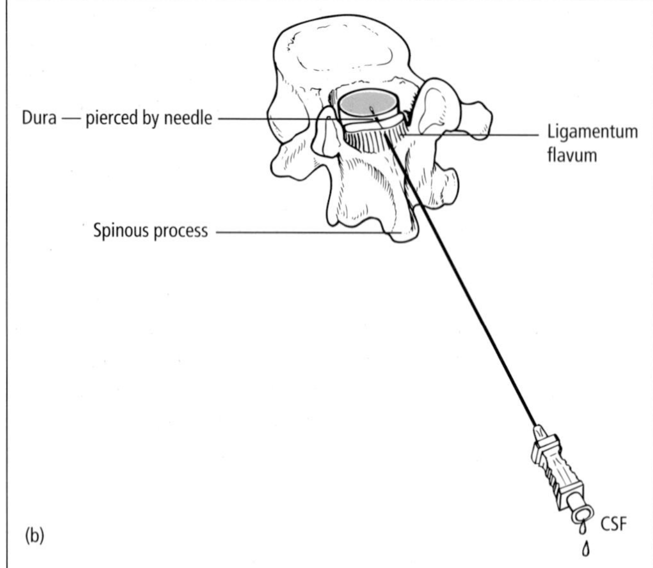

Figure 3.12 (a) Placement of the needle tip for epidural anaesthesia. (b) Placement of the needle tip for spinal (intrathecal) anaesthesia. From Gwinnutt CL *Clinical Anaesthesia*. Oxford: Blackwell Science, 1996.

quality and duration of analgesia, for example fentanyl 50 μg. For details of infusions of local anaesthetics and opioids for postoperative analgesia, see page 104.

Spinal anaesthesia

Spinal (intrathecal) anaesthesia results from the injection of a local anaesthetic drug directly into the cerebrospinal fluid (CSF), within the subarachnoid space (Fig. 3.12b). The spinal needle can only be inserted below the second lumbar and above the first sacral vertebrae; the upper limit is determined by the termination of the spinal cord, and the lower limit by the fact that the sacral vertebrae are fused and access becomes virtually impossible. A single injection of local anaesthetic is usually used, thereby limiting the duration of the technique.

A fine, 22–29 gauge, needle with a 'pencil point' or tapered point (e.g. Whitacre or Sprotte needle) is used (Fig. 3.13). The small diameter and shape are an attempt to reduce the incidence of postdural puncture headache (see below). To aid passage of this needle through the skin and interspinous ligament, a short, wide-bore needle is introduced initially and the spinal needle passed through its lumen.

Factors influencing the spread of the local anaesthetic drug within the CSF, and hence the extent of anaesthesia, include:

- Use of hyperbaric solutions (i.e. its specific gravity is greater than that of the CSF), for example 'heavy' bupivacaine (0.5%). This is achieved by the addition of 8% dextrose. Posture is then used to control spread.
- Positioning of the patient either during or after the injection. Maintenance of the sitting position after injection results in a block of the low lumbar and sacral nerves. In the supine position, the block will extend to the thoracic nerves around T5–T6, the point of maximum backwards curve (kyphosis) of the thoracic spine. Further extension can be obtained with a head-down tilt.
- Increasing the dose (volume and/or concentration) of local anaesthetic drug.
- The higher the placement of the spinal anaesthetic in the lumbar region, the higher the level of block obtained.

Small doses of an opioid, for example morphine or diamorphine 0.1–0.25 mg, may be injected with the local anaesthetic. This extends the duration of analgesia for up to 12–24 h postoperatively.

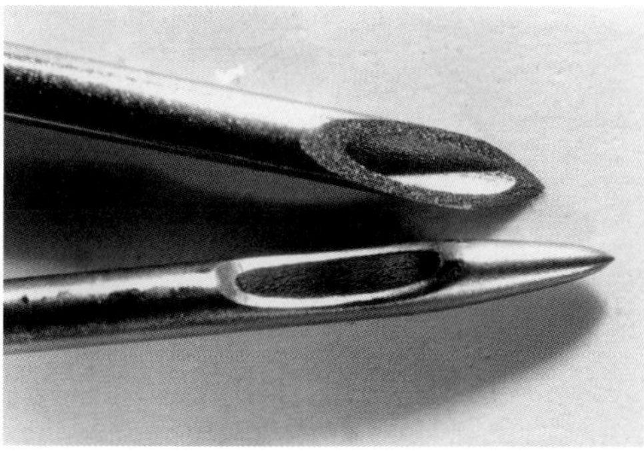

Figure 3.13 Photomicrograph showing the shape of a bevel needle (*top*) and 'pencil point' needle (*below*). Courtesy of the *British Journal of Radiology* 1994.

Contraindications to epidural and spinal anaesthesia

- *Hypovolaemia*: as a result of either blood loss or dehydration. Such patients are likely to experience severe falls in cardiac output as compensatory vasoconstriction is lost.
- *A low, fixed cardiac output*: as seen with severe aortic or mitral stenosis. The reduced venous return further reduces cardiac output, jeopardizing perfusion of vital organs.
- *Local skin sepsis*: risk of introducing infection.
- *Coagulopathy*: as a result of either a bleeding diathesis (e.g. haemophilia) or therapeutic anticoagulation. This risks causing an epidural haematoma. There may also be a very small risk in patients taking aspirin and associated drugs which reduce platelet activity. Where heparins are used perioperatively to reduce the risk of DVT, these may be started after the insertion of the epidural or spinal.
- *Raised intracranial pressure*: risk of precipitating coning.
- *Known allergy to amide local anaesthetic drugs.*
- A patient who is totally uncooperative.
- Concurrent disease of the CNS: some would caution against the use of these techniques for fear of being blamed for any subsequent deterioration.
- Previous spinal surgery or abnormal spinal anatomy: although not an absolute contraindication, epidural or spinal anaesthesia may be technically difficult.

Monitoring during local and regional anaesthesia

During epidural and spinal anaesthesia, the guidelines on monitoring (see page 28) should be followed. A conscious patient is not an excuse for inadequate monitoring! Particular attention must be paid to the cardiovascular system as a result of the profound effects these techniques can have. Maintenance of verbal contact with the patient is useful as it gives an indication of cerebral perfusion. Early signs of inadequate

Table 3.4 Incidence of common complications with spinal anaesthesia.

Hypotension	33%
Nausea	18%
Bradycardia	13%
Vomiting	7%
Arrhythmias	2%
Postdural puncture headache	<1%

cardiac output are complaints of nausea and faintness, and subsequent vomiting. The first indication of extensive spread of anaesthesia may be a complaint of difficulty with breathing or numbness in the fingers. Clearly, these valuable signs and symptoms will be lost if the patient is heavily sedated.

Complications of central neural blockade

These are usually mild and rarely cause any lasting morbidity (Table 3.4). Those commonly seen intraoperatively are predominantly due to the effects of the local anaesthetic. Their management is covered below. Complications seen in patients receiving epidural analgesia postoperatively are covered on Chapter 4, page 105.

Hypotension and bradycardia

Anaesthesia of the lumbar and thoracic nerves causes progressive sympathetic block, leading to vasodilatation and a reduction in the peripheral resistance and venous return to the heart and fall in cardiac output. If the block extends cranially beyond T5, the cardioaccelerator nerves are also blocked, and the unopposed vagal tone results in a bradycardia. Small falls in blood pressure are tolerated and may be helpful in reducing blood loss. If the blood pressure falls more than 25% of resting value, or the patient becomes symptomatic (see below), treatment consists of:

- oxygen via a facemask;
- IV fluids (crystalloids or colloids) to increase venous return;
- vasopressors to counteract the vasodilatation, either ephedrine, an alpha- and beta-agonist (3 mg IV), or metaraminol, an alpha-agonist (0.25 mg IV);
- atropine 0.5 mg IV to counteract bradycardia.

Nausea and vomiting

These are most often the first indications of hypotension and cerebral hypoxia, but can also result from vagal stimulation during upper abdominal surgery. Any hypotension or hypoxia is corrected as described above. If due to surgery, try to reduce the degree of manipulation. If this is not possible, then it may be necessary to convert to general anaesthesia. Atropine 0.3–0.6 mg is frequently effective, particularly if there is a bradycardia. Antiemetics can be tried (e.g. metoclopramide 10 mg IV), but this must not be at the expense of the above.

Postdural puncture headache

Caused by a persistent leak of CSF from the needle hole in the lumbar dura. The incidence is greatest with large holes, i.e. when a hole is made accidentally during epidural anaesthesia, and least after spinal anaesthesia using fine needles (e.g. 26 gauge) with a pencil or tapered point (<1%). Patients usually complain of a headache that is frontal or occipital, postural, and exacerbated by straining. The majority will resolve spontaneously. Persistent headaches can be relieved (>90%) by injecting 20–30 mL of the patient's own venous blood into the epidural space (epidural blood patch) under strict aseptic conditions.

Local anaesthetic toxicity

This is usually the result of one of the following:

- *Rapid absorption of a normally safe dose* Use of an excessively concentrated solution or injection into a vascular area results in rapid absorption. It can also occur during IVRA (see below) if the tourniquet is released too soon or accidentally.
- *Inadvertent IV injection* Failure to aspirate prior to injection via virtually any route.
- *Administration of an overdose* Failure or error in either calculating the maximum safe dose or taking

into account any pre-existing cardiac or hepatic disease.

Signs and symptoms of toxicity are due to effects on the CNS and the cardiovascular system. These are dependent on the plasma concentration and initially may represent either a mild toxicity or, more significantly, the early stages of a more severe reaction.

- *Mild or early*: circumoral paraesthesia, numbness of the tongue, visual disturbances, lightheadedness, slurred speech, twitching, restlessness, mild hypotension, and bradycardia.
- *Severe or late*: grand mal convulsions followed by coma, respiratory depression, and eventually apnoea, cardiovascular collapse with profound hypotension and bradycardia, and, ultimately, cardiac arrest.

Management of toxicity

If a patient complains of any of the above symptoms or exhibits signs, stop giving the local anaesthetic immediately! The next steps consist of:

- *Airway* Maintain using basic techniques. Tracheal intubation will be needed if the protective reflexes are absent to protect against aspiration.
- *Breathing* Give oxygen (100%) with support of ventilation if inadequate.
- *Circulation* Raise the patient's legs to encourage venous return and start an IV infusion of crystalloid or colloid. Treat a bradycardia with IV atropine. If no major pulse is palpable, start external cardiac compression. Give 100 ml bolus Intralipid® 20% over 1 min. If inotropes and vasopressors are required, invasive monitoring will be needed, and this should be performed on the ICU.
- *Convulsions* These must be treated early. Diazepam 5–10 mg IV can be used initially, but this may cause significant respiratory depression. If the convulsions do not respond or they recur, then seek assistance.

Because of the risk of an inadvertent overdose of a local anaesthetic drug, they should only be given where full facilities for monitoring and resuscitation are immediately available. In this way the patient will recover without any permanent sequelae.

Regional anaesthesia, awake or after induction of anaesthesia?

Major nerve blocks and epidural anaesthesia are often combined with general anaesthesia to reduce the amount and number of systemic drugs given, and to provide postoperative analgesia.

Claimed advantages of performing the block with the patient awake

- The block can be checked before surgery commences to ensure it works satisfactorily.
- The risk of nerve injury is reduced as the patient will complain if the needle touches a nerve.
- The patient can cooperate with positioning.

Claimed advantages of performing the block after induction of anaesthesia

- It is more pleasant for the patient, with no discomfort during insertion of the needle.
- There is no risk of the patient suddenly moving.
- It allows easier positioning of patients in pain, for example due to fractures.
- If the needle hits the nerve then the damage has already been done.

Fortunately, in experienced hands with either technique, the risk of nerve injury resulting in permanent sequelae is very rare. However, all patients who have a regional technique should be assessed to ensure that there is full recovery of normal function.

Transfer into the operating theatre

All of the above takes place in the anaesthetic room. At some point the patient has to be transferred into the operating theatre. This may take place with the patient already in position and on the operating table, or they may be taken into theatre on a trolley and then transferred on to the operating table. In either case, it will often mean disconnecting the patient from the anaesthesia machine and monitoring.

Once in theatre, the first manoeuvre must be to connect the patient to the breathing circuit and ensure that they are breathing or being ventilated adequately with an appropriate gas mixture. If not already on the operating table they are then transferred and the remaining monitoring attached. Every time a move has been completed it is essential to ensure that the airway is not compromised and ventilation maintained.

Positioning the patient

The patient is placed in a position to facilitate surgical access and there must always be sufficient theatre staff available to achieve this task safely, for both the patient and themselves. Some positions will require additional equipment; this must be assembled before any movement of the patient begins. The overall positioning is carried out under the direction and with the assistance of the anaesthetist. At all times the prime concern remains the safety of the patient. Detailed adjustment is carried out in conjunction with the surgeon.

The supine position (Fig. 3.14)

This position is used for the majority of surgical operations, but there is no room for complacency. The patient lies flat on their back, with the head and neck in a neutral position, unless the surgeon requires otherwise, for example surgery to the ear. The arms are placed alongside the patient's sides or flexed at the elbow lying across the lower chest. If an arm or hand is to be operated on, this limb is usually abducted and supported on an arm table. The legs are extended in a neutral position.

In this position, the abdominal contents push the diaphragm into the thorax, reducing the lung volume (FRC). There is also the tendency for dependent alveoli to be better perfused but not as well ventilated. The overall effect is to reduce oxygenation of the blood, but this is compensated for by increasing the inspired oxygen concentration to a minimum of 30%

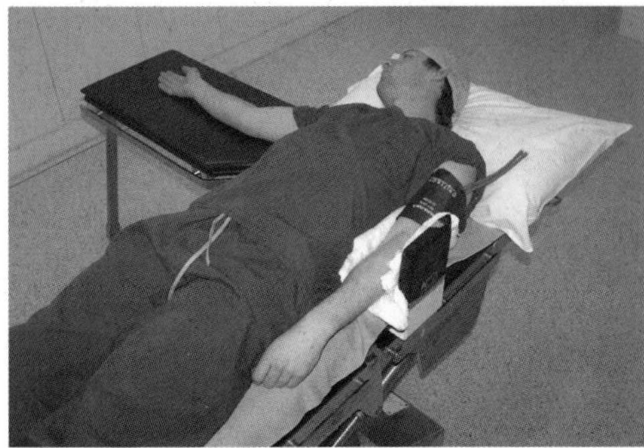

Figure 3.14 Supine position.

Points to note:

- The radial nerve is at risk from pressure midway along the humerus from a misplaced arm retainer.
- The ulnar nerve can be damaged at the elbow if allowed to lie over the edge of the mattress.
- The median nerve can be damaged in the antecubutal fossa by the distal edge of the blood pressure cuff if the elbow is flexed excessively.
- The common peroneal nerve can be damaged by pressure against the head of the fibula.
- The head should be turned towards an abducted arm to reduce traction on the ipsilateral brachial plexus.
- Pneumatic calf compression devices are used to reduce venous stasis in the legs and risk of DVT.

Variations in the supine position

- *Trendelenburg*: head-down, using gravity to help displace bowels from the pelvis. Used in gynaecological and pelvic surgery.
- *Lithotomy*: with the hips and knees flexed to 90°, legs abducted slightly, and the ankles supported in stirrups. Extremes of flexion and rotation must be avoided as the sciatic and femoral nerves can be damaged. The deep calf veins can be compressed against the stirrup poles. Used in gynaecological, urological, and anorectal surgery.
- *Lloyd-Davies*: hips and knees flexed 30–40°, abducted, and supported in gutters. This position is designed to allow the surgical team combined access to the abdomen and perineum.

The lateral position (Fig. 3.15)

This is a relatively unstable position and requires a variety of additional supports to ensure the

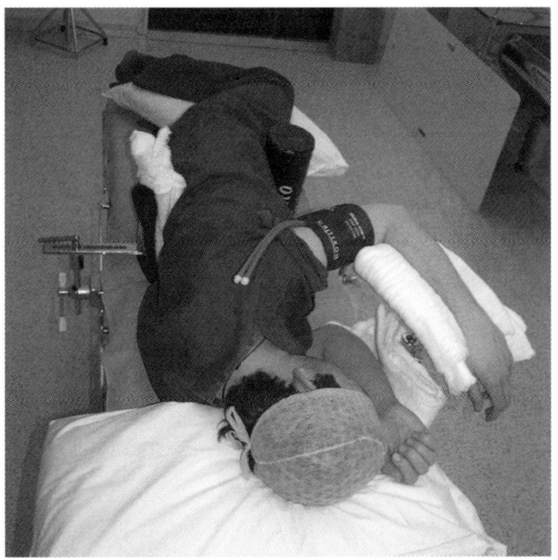

Figure 3.15 Lateral position.

patient's safety. The anaesthetist takes responsibility for the patient's head and neck (and airway), and coordinates the team as the patient is turned. Depending on the site of surgery (chest, abdomen (flank), or hip), supports are placed posteriorly against the pelvis, lumbar or thoracic spine, and anteriorly against the iliac crests. The upper arm is usually supported in a small gutter, again the exact position depending on the site of surgery, and the lower arm is placed to lie either across the chest or adjacent to the head, flexed at the shoulder and elbow.

In this position, during mechanical ventilation, the upper lung will be preferentially ventilated while the lower lung will receive a relatively greater blood flow. This can adversely affect oxygenation, particularly in patients with pre-existing pulmonary disease. More invasive monitoring may be used in this position.

Points to note:

- The patient's head and neck are supported to prevent traction on the brachial plexus on the uppermost side, and a small support placed in the dependent axilla to prevent traction on the plexus on the patient's lower side.
- Ensure that the patient's lower ear is not folded back on itself.
- Care when turning the patient to ensure that intravascular cannulae, tracheal tube, and urinary catheter are not caught and removed.

The prone position (Fig. 3.16)

Many variations in this position have evolved using specially designed supports. Only the basic prone position will be described here.

As described above, the anaesthetist takes control of the head and neck and coordinates the team. With their arms kept at their sides, the patient is turned in two stages: first into the lateral position, and then prone. It is essential that turning the patient does not leave them flat on the table; either

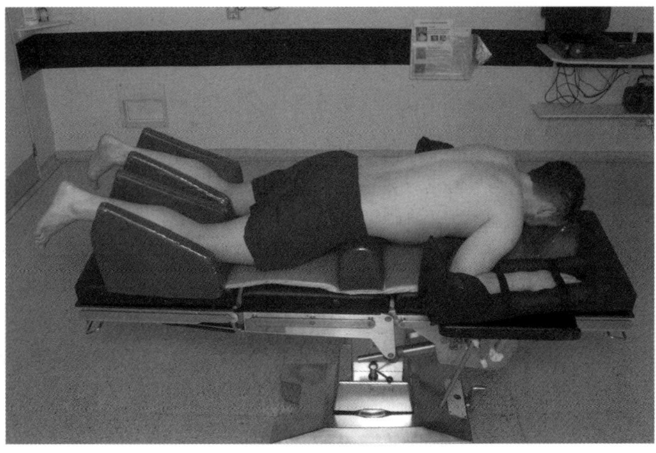

Figure 3.16 Prone position.

the head end of the table is lowered or the body is raised to prevent excessive extension of the head and neck. Supports are required beneath the chest and pelvis, ensuring that the abdomen is free and the femoral vessels are not under undue pressure. The head must be supported in such a way as to prevent pressure on the eyes or tip of the nose, or occlusion of the tracheal tube. The patient's arms are either retained at their sides or flexed at the elbow and abducted at the shoulder to lie adjacent to their head. Finally, the knees are slightly flexed and padding is placed beneath the shins to raise the toes.

This position has the least detrimental effect on respiratory function. Ventilation and perfusion remain well matched, minimizing the risk of hypoxaemia. One of the main risks is obstruction of the inferior vena cava from badly placed supports reducing venous return, cardiac output, and blood pressure. Careful checks must be made after turning the patient and close monitoring of the cardiovascular system is essential.

Points to note:

- A reinforced tracheal tube is used to reduce the risk of the tube kinking. This would be difficult to correct once prone.
- Great care must be taken with the cervical spine in ALL patients to prevent excessive rotation or extension.
- The arms must never be forced into position against resistance; the neck of the humerus is easily fractured.
- Pressure on the eyes may cause thrombosis of the retinal artery and blindness.
- Avoid compression of the femoral vessels in the groin; check the capillary refill time and colour of the feet after turning.
- Ensure that pressure is not applied to the male genitalia by badly placed pelvic supports.
- Avoid traction on the sciatic nerve by slightly flexing the knees.
- The abdomen must be free, particularly in spinal surgery, as compression of the inferior vena cava will divert blood via the epidural veins that may compromise spinal surgery by excessive bleeding.

One of the most common reasons for turning a surgical patient prone is to operate on their spine. This may be the result of degenerative disease processes or trauma that may restrict movement. As the patient will have normally been given neuromuscular blocking drugs, it is very easy to inflict damage to the spinal cord either by placing the patient in an unsafe position or by uncontrolled movement when they are turned; the cervical spine is particularly susceptible.

Keeping patients warm

Most patients' core temperature falls during anaesthesia as a result of exposure to a cold environment, evaporation of fluids from body cavities, the administration of cold IV fluids, and breathing dry, cold anaesthetic gases. This is compounded by the loss of body temperature regulation and inability to shiver. These can be minimized by forced air warming, a process in which warm air is blown over the surface of the patient that is not exposed for surgery via a perforated blanket. In addition, all fluids (particularly blood) are warmed to body temperature, inspired gases are warmed and humidified, and all other exposed areas covered.

Assessment of neuromuscular blockade

The electrodes of the nerve stimulator can be applied to either the facial nerve just in front if the tragus or over the ulnar nerve at the wrist. A variety of sequences of electrical stimulation can be used to assess the intensity of neuromuscular block. This is useful during long surgical procedures to control the timing of increments or adjust the rate of an infusion of neuromuscular blocking drugs to prevent coughing or sudden movement. This is particularly important during surgery in which a microscope is used, for example neurosurgery. At the end of surgery, it allows the anaesthetist to plan reversal of residual neuromuscular block to ensure adequate respiratory muscle function. It is also used to differentiate between apnoea due to prolonged action of suxamethonium, suggesting pseudocholinesterase deficiency, and residual non-depolarizing block, when both have been given. Finally, in recovery, the use of a nerve stimulator will allow the anaesthetist to distinguish between residual neuromuscular block and opioid overdose as a cause of inadequate ventilation postoperatively. The former will show reduced or absent response to stimulation, the latter a normal response.

Intraoperative fluids

The type and volume of fluid given during surgery vary for each and every patient, but must take into account:

- any deficit the patient has accrued;
- intraoperative requirements;
- maintenance requirements during the procedure;
- losses due to surgery;
- any vasodilatation secondary to the use of a regional anaesthetic technique (see page 72).

The accrued deficit

This may be due to preoperative fasting, or losses as a result of vomiting, haemorrhage, or pyrexia. Any deficit due to fasting is predominantly water from the total body water volume. The volume required is calculated at the normal daily maintenance rate of 1.5 mL/kg/h (from the point at which fasting began). Although this deficit can be replaced with a fluid such as 4% glucose plus 0.18% saline, Hartmann's solution is widely used intraoperatively. The other main cause of a preoperative deficit is losses either from or into the gastrointestinal tract. This fluid usually contains electrolytes and effectively depletes the extracellular volume. It is best replaced with a crystalloid of similar composition, particularly in respect of the sodium concentration, for example 0.9% sodium chloride or Hartmann's solution.

Acute blood loss preoperatively can be replaced with either an appropriate volume of crystalloid (remembering that only 30% remains intravascular) or colloid. If more than 30% of the estimated blood volume has been lost (approximately 1500 mL), and bleeding is ongoing, blood should be used.

Intraoperative requirements

Maintenance fluids are usually given when surgery is prolonged (along with any accrued deficit), or if there is the possibility of a delay in the patient resuming oral fluid intake. Most patients will compensate for a preoperative deficit by increasing their oral intake postoperatively. When maintenance fluid is used it should be given at 1.5 mL/kg/h, and increased if the patient is pyrexial by 10% for each degree centigrade above normal.

Losses during surgery are due to:

- *Evaporation* This can occur during body cavity surgery or when large areas of tissue are exposed, depleting the total body water.
- *Trauma* Leads to the formation of tissue oedema, the volume of which is dependent upon the extent of tissue damage, and is similar in composition to ECF. This fluid is often referred to as 'third space loss' (see Chapter 4) and creates a deficit in their ECF volume that can no longer be accessed.
- *Blood loss* This will depend upon the type and site of surgery.

Fluid losses from the first two causes are difficult to measure and are extremely variable. If evaporative losses are considered excessive, then 4% glucose plus 0.18% saline can be used. Third space losses should be replaced with a solution similar in composition to ECF, and Hartmann's is commonly used. The rate of administration and volume required is proportional to surgical trauma and may be as much as 10 mL/kg/h. Blood pressure, pulse, peripheral perfusion, and urine output will give an indication as to the adequacy of replacement, but in complex cases where there are other causes of fluid loss, particularly bleeding, the trend of the CVP is very useful.

Blood loss is slightly more obvious and can be estimated by weighing surgical swabs and noting the volume in the suction apparatus (minus the volume of any saline washes used). Most previously well patients will tolerate the anaemia that results from the loss of 30% of their blood volume, providing that the circulating volume is adequately maintained by the use of crystalloids or colloids. Beyond this, red cell preparations are used in order to maintain the oxygen-carrying capacity of the blood. A haemoglobin level between 8 and 10 g/dL is safe even for those patients with serious cardiorespiratory disease. In most cases, the equivalent of the patient's estimated blood volume can be replaced with red cell concentrates, crystalloid, and colloid in the appropriate volumes. Occasionally, blood loss is such that the haemostatic mechanisms are affected. This may be seen as continuous oozing from the surgical wound or around IV cannulation sites. If this is suspected, the patient's coagulation status must be assessed by platelet count, prothrombin time (PT) or international normalized ratio (INR), and fibrinogen levels. Platelets may not be required until blood loss exceeds 1.5 times the estimated blood volume. Treatment is usually reserved for those cases in which the INR reaches 1.7–2.0, the fibrinogen levels fall below 0.5 g/L, or the platelet count falls below 50×10^9/L.

The anaesthetic record

On every occasion an anaesthetic is administered, a comprehensive and *legible* record must be made. The details and method of recording will vary with each case, the type of chart used, and the equipment available. The anaesthetic record is valuable to future anaesthetists who encounter the patient, particularly when there has been a difficulty (e.g. with intubation), and is also a medicolegal document, which may be referred to after several years. An anaesthetic chart typically allows the following to be recorded:

- preoperative findings, ASA grade, premedication;
- details of previous anaesthetics and any difficulties;
- apparatus used for the current anaesthetic;
- monitoring devices used;
- anaesthetic and other drugs administered: timing, dose, and route;
- vital signs at various intervals, usually depicted graphically;
- fluids administered and lost: type and volume;
- use of local or regional anaesthetic techniques;
- anaesthetic difficulties or complications;
- postoperative instructions.

Increasingly, electronic records are being developed. These have the advantage of allowing the anaesthetist to concentrate on caring for the patient, particularly during an emergency, rather than having to stop and make a record or try to fill in the record retrospectively.

Recovery from anaesthesia

At the end of surgery, the anaesthetist has to reverse the process of anaesthesia, often referred to as 'waking the patient up'. If only it was that simple! As a consequence of the wide variety of anaesthetic techniques used, there is no absolute protocol for this stage of anaesthesia. However, there are two main priorities: recovery of consciousness and maintenance of a patent airway. Here, these will be described in relation to patients breathing spontaneously and those being ventilated.

Spontaneous ventilation, inhalational drug for maintenance, and laryngeal mask airway

At the end of surgery, the vaporizer is turned off and the patient allowed to eliminate the inhaled anaesthetic. If a circle system is being used, the patient will continue to rebreathe the exhaled gas. This will contain some anaesthetic agent and so the alveolar, and hence plasma, concentrations will only fall very slowly, delaying recovery. Therefore, to speed up elimination of the anaesthetic, the flow of oxygen into the circle is increased to around 10–15 L/min. This excess flow flushes exhaled gas out of the circle, rebreathing is eliminated, and the inspired oxygen concentration is almost 100%. The LMA will now need to be removed. There are two options as to when this is done:

- Remove while deeply unconscious. This is easier but leaves the airway unprotected, and the lack of muscle tone may result in airway obstruction and the need for the anaesthetist to perform a chin lift or jaw thrust.
- Leave the LMA in place with the patient breathing oxygen until they are almost fully conscious. By this time, the patient's muscle tone, and ability to protect their airway will be restored, but may result in the patient biting on the tube and obstructing the airway.

Once the LMA has been removed, oxygen is given via a facemask, and if not already carried out the patient is transferred from the operating table to a trolley. As the patient begins to obey commands, they can be sat up at 30° if it is safe to do so.

Mechanical ventilation, inhalational drug for maintenance, and tracheal tube

The main difference from what has already been described is that normal neuromuscular function has to be restored before the patient regains consciousness. Therefore, recovery needs to be coordinated with the point at which the neuromuscular blocking drug wears off spontaneously or is antagonized. This is best checked by using a peripheral nerve stimulator. As before, the fresh gas flow is increased and the patient ventilated with 100% oxygen to eliminate the volatile drug. If necessary, a dose of neostigmine (2.5 mg) is given to antagonize the effect of the neuromuscular blocker given along with an anticholinergic, usually glycopyrrolate, to block the unwanted muscarinic effects of neostigmine. The aim is to restore spontaneous ventilation before removal of the tracheal tube. Once ventilation commences, a similar dilemma over when to remove the tube is encountered as before:

- Remove while deeply unconscious. This leaves the airway unprotected and at risk of obstruction, and the need for support by the anaesthetist or the use of an oropharyngeal airway. Furthermore, there is also the risk of the patient developing laryngospasm if any soiling of the larynx occurs (e.g. from saliva or regurgitated gastric contents) as the patient recovers.
- Leave in place until nearly conscious. Apart from the risk of occlusion by the patient biting the tube, the presence of the tube may also induce severe coughing and breath-holding by the patient. This may cause hypoxia, as well as being painful after abdominal surgery, and undesirable after intracranial surgery as it may precipitate bleeding.

When a TIVA technique has been used to maintain anaesthesia, the principles are the same, except that the infusions are stopped to allow the plasma concentration of drug to fall to promote diffusion out of the brain. When remifentanil has been used intraoperatively, the patient will need to be given an alternative analgesic before recovering to prevent them being in severe pain when they awaken.

Special circumstances

Anaesthesia for emergency surgery

It is assumed that patients who need anaesthetizing for emergency surgery will have a full stomach, and there is an increased risk of regurgitation and aspiration into the lungs. The greatest risk is during induction of anaesthesia, but some patients are also at risk during extubation and recovery. The incidence of complications appears to be related to both the volume (>25 mL) and pH (<2.5) of the material aspirated. Factors predisposing to aspiration include:

- *A full stomach*: an inadequate period of starvation (emergency patients), increased gastrointestinal contents secondary to bowel obstruction distension following facemask ventilation.
- *Delayed gastric emptying*: drugs (especially opiates), trauma (particularly head injury), peritoneal irritation, blood in the stomach, pain and anxiety.
- *Obstetric patients*.
- *Other causes*: a history of gastro-oesophageal reflux, hiatus hernia, obesity, head-down position, presence of a bulbar palsy, oesophageal pouch or stricture.

Consequently, in these patients, measures will be taken to prevent aspiration, and the majority will be intubated in order to secure and protect their airway. In order to achieve this as safely as possible, the technique used for induction of anaesthesia is slightly modified and referred to as rapid-sequence induction or RSI.

Prevention of aspiration

A variety of methods are used, alone or in combination:

1 Reduction of residual gastric volume:

- An adequate period of preoperative starvation.
- Avoidance of drugs that delay gastric emptying.

• Insertion of a nasogastric tube.
• Use of gastrokinetic drugs, for example metoclopramide.

2 Increase pH of gastric contents:
• Sodium citrate to neutralize gastric acid.
• H_2 antagonists, for example ranitidine.
• Proton pump inhibitors, for example omeprazole, and lansoprazole at the moment especially as there are the fastabs which dissolve under the tongue in patients NBM (nil by mouth) or unable to swallow.

3 Use of cricoid pressure (see below).

Cricoid pressure (Sellick's manoeuvre)

Aspiration of regurgitated gastric contents is a life-threatening complication of anaesthesia, and every effort must be made to minimize the risk. Cricoid pressure is used as a physical barrier to regurgitation in patients at high risk of regurgitation. The cricoid cartilage is the only complete ring of cartilage in the larynx, and pressure on its anterior aspect forces the whole ring posteriorly. This compresses the oesophagus against the body of the sixth cervical vertebra, occluding it and preventing regurgitation. The manoeuvre is carried out by an assistant, applying pressure as the patient loses consciousness using the thumb and index finger of their right hand whilst the other hand stabilizes the patient's neck from behind (Fig. 3.17). Cricoid pressure should be maintained even if the patient starts to actively vomit, as the risk of aspiration is greater than the theoretical risk of oesophageal rupture.

Rapid-sequence induction of anaesthesia

Preoxygenation is achieved as already described, during which time monitors are attached, venous access is secured if not already done, and an IV infusion started. The suction apparatus is switched on and a rigid Yankeur sucker attached and placed within immediate reach of the anaesthetist. A check is made that the anaesthetic assistant is able to apply cricoid pressure effectively and they understand it is not to be released until instruction is given by the anaesthetist to do so. The patient must also be warned that they will feel pressure on their neck as they lose consciousness.

When preoxygenation is judged to be adequate, the predetermined dose of the induction drug is given into a fast running IV infusion and, as consciousness is lost, cricoid pressure is applied and suxamethonium is given. The facemask is held against the patient's face, but manual ventilation is not performed. To do so would risk forcing oxygen into the stomach, distending it, and increase the risk of regurgitation. The patient is observed for the fasciculations caused by suxamethonium and, once they have stopped, direct laryngoscopy is performed and the patient intubated. The cuff of the tracheal tube is inflated and satisfactory position of

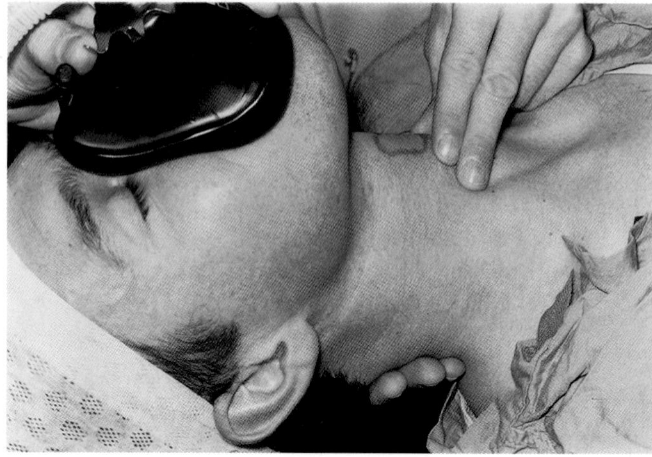

Figure 3.17 Cricoid pressure (Sellick's manoeuvre). Note the position of the thyroid cartilage marked on the patient's neck.

the tube confirmed as already described. Once the anaesthetist is confident that the tube is in the trachea, cricoid pressure is released.

Anaesthesia and surgery then continue as described previously, using either an inhalational or IV technique to maintain anaesthesia. A non-depolarizing neuromuscular blocking drug is given when there is evidence, either clinically or by using a nerve stimulator, that the effect of suxamethonium is diminishing. It is not unusual to pass a nasogastric (or orogastric) tube during anaesthesia to allow aspiration of gastric contents. However, this does not always guarantee complete emptying of the stomach. Therefore, at the end of surgery, whenever possible it is safer to extubate a patient on their side and leave them in this position until they have fully regained their laryngeal reflexes.

Anaesthesia for obstetric patients

Obstetric patients may require anaesthesia for a variety of surgical procedures, but the most common is for a caesarean section, either electively or as an emergency usually when the mother is already in labour. The following is an outline of the principles of anaesthesia.

There are three main anaesthetic techniques for a caesarean section: general, epidural, or spinal anaesthesia. The latter two can be performed together (combined spinal–epidural, CSE) but will not be covered further.

General anaesthesia is a rapid and reliable form of anaesthesia, but is less common now due to the increasing use of spinals and epidurals. There are a number of associated problems:

1 There is an increased risk of regurgitation and aspiration. This is due to the progesterone-induced relaxation of the lower oesophageal sphincter and increased intra-abdominal pressure from the presence of the gravid uterus. This is exacerbated by the fact that in labour, gastric emptying is very slow. All pregnant women requiring general anaesthesia are regarded as having a full stomach and receive antacid prophylaxis to increase the pH and reduce the volume of gastric contents, and anaesthesia is induced using an RSI as described above. During emergency surgery, a gastric tube is passed to try and empty the stomach, and patients should be extubated and recovered in the lateral position.

2 Failed intubation is more common in obstetric patients (1:250 compared with 1:2000 non-obstetric patients). This is primarily due to anatomical factors, in particular enlargement of breast tissue, fatty deposits in the airway, and the fact that most women have a full set of teeth. When combined with the fact that the FRC is reduced and oxygen consumption increased, the pregnant woman will desaturate and become hypoxic remarkably quickly during repeated attempts at intubation. Attention must be paid to ensuring full preoxygenation, head and neck position must be optimized, and intubation must only be attempted at the point of maximal action of suxamethonium. If intubation fails, institute a failed intubation drill. Oxygenation is more important than intubation.

3 Maternal awareness as a result of the use of inadequate doses of the induction and inhalational drugs in an attempt to avoid oversedating the baby. Adequate doses of drugs must be given; 'flat' babies can be resuscitated by a paediatrician.

Epidurals are predominantly used to provide analgesia during labour. The extent and intensity of the block can be increased (anaesthesia) to allow caesarean section to take place. However, this is a relatively slow process and there is a risk of inadequate anaesthesia due to inadequate or absent block of some nerve roots. The technique and other problems are as described above.

Spinal anaesthesia is now the choice for elective and most emergency caesarean sections, providing quick, reliable, and intense anaesthesia. The main problems associated with this technique are that unlike general and epidural anaesthesia, it is time limited, and hypotension is more common. Other complications are as described above. Increasingly, opioids are used along with the local anaesthetic drug to reduce the dose of the latter, and increase the effectiveness and duration to provide postoperative analgesia.

Aortocaval compression

As the gravid uterus enlarges through the pregnancy, it compresses the inferior vena cava, reducing venous return to the heart, cardiac output, and blood pressure. It is maximal at around 36 weeks gestation, worse in the supine position, and exacerbated by the sympathetic block produced by epidurals and spinals. In addition, compression of the aorta may occur, reducing blood pressure and flow in the uterine arteries that may cause foetal hypoxia. Both of these effects can be prevented by using a left lateral tilt in the supine patient, and it is essential that whichever technique of anaesthesia is used for a caesarean section, the mother is placed in this position.

Aspiration of gastric contents

Despite taking all of the precautions outlined above, occasionally regurgitation and aspiration still occur. Signs suggesting aspiration include:

- coughing during induction or recovery from anaesthesia, gastric contents in the pharynx at laryngoscopy, or around the edge of the facemask;
- if severe, there is progressive hypoxia, bronchospasm, and respiratory obstruction.

Occasionally, aspiration may go completely unnoticed during anaesthesia, with the development of hypoxia, hypotension, and respiratory failure postoperatively.

Management

- Maintain a patent airway and place the patient head-down and on his or her side, preferably the left; intubation is relatively easier on this side.
- Aspirate any material from the pharynx, preferably under direct vision (use a laryngoscope).

(i) Neuromuscular blocking drugs not given; surgery not urgent

- Give 100% oxygen via a facemask.
- Allow the patient to recover, give oxygen to maintain a satisfactory $Sp\text{O}_2$.
- Treat bronchospasm with salbutamol or ipratroprium as described on page 83.
- Take a chest X-ray and organize regular physiotherapy.
- Depending on degree of aspiration, consider monitoring on the ICU or HDU.

(ii) Neuromuscular blocking drugs not given; surgery essential

- Get help, empty the stomach with a nasogastric tube, and instil 30 mL of sodium citrate.
- After allowing the patient to recover, continue using either a regional technique or an RSI and intubation.
- After intubation, aspirate the tracheobronchial tree and consider bronchoscopy.
- Treat bronchospasm as above.
- Postoperatively, arrange for a chest X-ray and physiotherapy.
- Recover in the ICU or HDU with oxygen therapy.
- Postoperative ventilation may be required.

(iii) Neuromuscular blocking drugs given

- Intubate with a cuffed tracheal tube to secure the airway.
- Aspirate the tracheobronchial tree before starting positive pressure ventilation.
- Consider bronchopulmonary lavage with saline.
- Treat bronchospasm as above.
- Pass a nasogastric tube and empty the stomach.
- If the patient is stable (i.e. not hypoxic or hypotensive), surgery can be continued with postoperative care as described above.

If oxygen saturation remains low despite 100% oxygen, consider the possibility of obstruction and the need for fibreoptic bronchoscopy.

If aspiration is suspected in a patient postoperatively, treat as for (i) above.

There is no place for routine administration of large-dose steroids. Antibiotics should be given according to local protocols. Unless surgery is potentially life-saving, those patients with bronchospasm resistant to treatment, or with persistent hypoxia or hypotension, should be transferred to the ICU for ventilation, with additional, invasive cardiorespiratory monitoring as needed.

Anaphylaxis

Most drug reactions in anaesthesia are mild and transient, consisting mainly of localized urticaria as a result of cutaneous histamine release. The incidence of anaphylaxis caused by anaesthetic drugs is between 1 : 10 000 and 1 : 20 000 drug administrations, and is more common in females. Of those reported to the Medicines Control Agency, 10% involved a fatality compared with 3.7% for drugs overall. This probably reflects the frequency with which anaesthetic drugs are given IV. Clinical features include (in order of frequency):

- severe hypotension;
- severe bronchospasm;
- widespread flushing;
- hypoxaemia;
- urticaria;
- angioedema, which may involve the airway;
- pruritus, nausea, and vomiting.

Cardiovascular collapse is the most common and severe feature. Asthmatics often develop bronchospasm that is resistant to treatment, and any circumstance that reduce the patient's catecholamine response (e.g. beta-blockers, spinal anaesthesia) will increase the severity.

Anaphylaxis involves the degranulation of cells and basophils as a result of , either an allergic (IgE-mediated) or non-allergic (non-IgE-mediated) reaction, liberating histamine, 5-HT, and associated vasoactive substances. The term anaphylactoid is no longer used. The European Academy of Allergology and Clinical Immunology Nomenclature Committee have proposed the following broad definition:

> 'Anaphylaxis is a severe, life-threatening generalized or systemic hypersensitivity reaction'.

Causes of allergic reactions

- *Anaesthetic drugs*:
  - muscle relaxants (>50%): suxamethonium, atracurium, rocuronium, vecuronium;
  - induction agents (5%): thiopentone, propofol.
- *Antibiotics (8%)*:
  - penicillin (<1% of patients may cross-react to modern cephalosporins).
- *IV fluids*:
  - colloids (3%), Haemacel, Gelofusine.
- Latex (17%).

Immediate management

- Discontinue all drugs likely to have triggered the reaction.
- Call for help.
- Maintain a patent airway, administer 100% oxygen, elevate the patient's legs providing ventilation is not compromised.
- Give adrenaline, 50 μg *slowly* IV (0.5 mL of 1 : 10 000) under ECG control. A dilution of 1 : 100 000 adrenaline (10 μg/mL) allows better titration and reduces the risk of adverse effects. If no ECG is available, give 0.5 mg IM (0.5 mL of 1 : 1000). If there is no improvement within 5 min, give a further dose.
- Give high flow oxygen, 10–15 L/min.
- Ensure adequate ventilation:
  - Intubation will be required if spontaneous ventilation is inadequate or in the presence of severe bronchospasm. This may be exceedingly difficult in the presence of severe laryngeal oedema. In these circumstances, a needle cricothyroidotomy or surgical airway will be required.
- Support the circulation:
  - Start a rapid IV infusion of fluids 10–20 mL/kg. Crystalloids initially may be safer than colloids. In the absence of a major pulse, start cardiopulmonary resuscitation using the protocol for pulseless electrical activity (PEA).
- Monitoring:
  - ECG, oxygenation of the peripheral tissues (SpO_2), blood pressure, end-tidal CO_2. Establish an arterial line and check the blood gases. Monitor CVP and urine output to assess adequacy of circulating volume.

Subsequent management

- *Antihistamines*: chlorphenamine (H_1 blocker) 10–20 mg slowly IV or IM . There is no evidence for the use of H_2 blockers.
- *Steroids*: hydrocortisone 200 mg slowly IV or IM. Helps stop late sequelae.
- *Bronchodilators*: salbutamol, 2.5–5.0 mg nebulized or 0.25 mg IV, ipratropium, 500 μg, or magnesium 2 g (8 mmol) slowly IV may be useful when there are severe, asthma-like features or if the

patient is taking beta-blockers. Magnesium may cause flushing and may worsen hypotension.

As soon as possible these patients should be transferred to an ICU for further treatment and monitoring. Reactions vary in severity, can be biphasic, delayed in onset (particularly latex sensitivity), and prolonged. An infusion of adrenaline may be required. The possibility of a tension pneumothorax (secondary to barotrauma) causing hypotension must not be forgotten.

Investigations

The most informative is measurement of plasma tryptase. A blood sample should be taken immediately after treatment and repeated approximately 1 and 6 h after the event. Elevated tryptase confirms that the reaction was associated with mast cell degranulation, but does not distinguish between an allergic and non-allergic cause. A negative test does not completely exclude anaphylaxis. Expert advice about follow-up and identification of the cause must be arranged.

Finally, record all details in the patient's notes, and do not forget to inform the patient and the patient's general practitioner of the events, both verbally and in writing. In the UK, report adverse drug events to the Medicines and Healthcare products Regulatory Agency by completing a 'yellow card' found in the BNF.

Generalized atopy does not help predict the risk of an immunologically mediated reaction to anaesthetic drugs. A previous history of 'allergy to an anaesthetic' is cause for concern, and there is a high risk of cross-reactivity between drugs of the same group. These patients must be investigated appropriately.

Malignant hyperpyrexia (hyperthermia)

This is a rare inherited disorder of skeletal muscle metabolism in which there is a release of abnormally high concentrations of calcium from the sarcoplasmic reticulum causing increased muscle activity and metabolism. Excess heat production causes a rise in core temperature of at least 2°C/h. It is triggered by exposure to the inhalational anaesthetic agents, halothane being the most potent, and suxamethonium. It is associated with surgery for squints, hernia repair, cleft palate repair, and orthopaedic surgery. The incidence is between 1:10 000 and 1:40 000 anaesthetized patients

Presentation

- A progressive rise in body temperature (may go unnoticed unless the patient's temperature is being monitored).
- An unexplained tachycardia.
- An increased end-tidal CO_2.
- Tachypnoea in spontaneously breathing patients.
- Muscle rigidity, failure to relax after suxamethonium, especially persistent masseter spasm.
- Cardiac arrhythmias.
- A falling oxygen saturation and cyanosis.

Immediate management

- GET HELP.
- Stop all anaesthetic agents, hyperventilate with 100% oxygen.
- Change the anaesthesia machine and circuits.
- Terminate surgery as soon as practical.
- Monitor core temperature.
- Give dantrolene 1 mg/kg IV (up to 10 mg/kg may be needed).
- Start active cooling:
  - cold 0.9% saline IV;
  - expose the patient completely;
  - surface cooling—ice over axillary and femoral arteries, wet sponging, and fanning to encourage cooling by evaporation;
  - consider gastric or peritoneal lavage with cold saline.
- Treat acidosis with 8.4% sodium bicarbonate in 50 mmol (50 mL) aliquots IV titrated to acid–base results:
- Treat hyperkalaemia.
- Transfer the patient to the ICU as soon as possible for:

- ○ temperature monitoring; may be labile for up to 48 h;
- ○ continue dantrolene to alleviate muscle rigidity;
- ○ monitor urine output for myoglobin and treat to prevent renal failure;
- ○ treatment of coagulopathy.

Dantrolene

The specific treatment for MH. Inhibits calcium release, inhibiting excitation–contraction and preventing further muscle activity. Dantrolene is orange in colour, supplied in vials containing 20 mg (plus 3 g of mannitol), requires 60 mL of water for reconstitution, and is very slow to dissolve.

Investigation of the family

Following an episode, the patient and their family should be referred to an MH Unit for investigation of their susceptibility to MH.

Anaesthesia for MH-susceptible patients

- Employ a regional technique using plain bupivacaine.
- General anaesthesia:
  - ○ use a designated vapour-free machine, new circuits and hoses;
  - ○ propofol, thiopentone, opioids, atracurium, and vecuronium are thought to be safe;
  - ○ a total IV technique using an infusion of propofol and remifentanil, with oxygen-enriched air for ventilation;
  - ○ consider pretreatment with dantrolene (orally or IV) in those who have survived a previous episode;
  - ○ monitor temperature; ensure cooling is available.

Useful websites

http://www.aagbi.org/publications/guidelines/docs/anaesthesiateam05.pdf

[The anaesthesia team. Revised edition 2005. The Association of Anaesthetists of Great Britain & Ireland.]

http://www.aagbi.org/publications/guidelines/docs/checking04.pdf

[Checking anaesthetic equipment. The Association of Anaesthetists of Great Britain & Ireland. 2004.]

http://anestit.unipa.it/HomePage.html

[The best anaesthesia site on the Web, with free sign-on, and a virtual textbook of anaesthesia that includes a good section on airway management.]

http://www.das.uk.com/

[The Difficult Airway Society website contains guidance on management of airway emergencies including failed intubation drills.]

http://www.nysora.com/

[The best regional anaesthesia website.]

www.oaa-anaes.ac.uk/

[The Obstetric Anaesthetists' Association website.]

http://www.resus.org.uk/pages/reaction.pdf

[Resuscitation Council UK. Emergency Treatment of Anaphylactic Reactions Guidelines for healthcase providers. January 2008.]

http://www.aagbi.org/publications/guidelines/docs/malignanthyp07.pdf

[The Association of Anaesthetists of Great Britain & Ireland guidelines for treatment of malignant hyperthermia. 2007.]

http://www.aagbi.org/publications/guidelines/docs/latoxicity07.pdf

[The Association of Anaesthetists of Great Britain & Ireland. Guidelines for the Management of Severe Local Anaesthetic Toxicity. 2007.]

All websites last accessed April 2008.

Self-assessment

3.1 What are the main advantages and disadvantages of inhalational induction of anaesthesia?

3.2 List in order of reliability the checks that can be performed to confirm the position of a tracheal tube. Give five common complications of tracheal intubation.

3.3 Give an example of a total intravenous anaesthetic technique (TIVA) in a patient undergoing a laparotomy. Give four each of potential advantages and disadvantages of this technique.

3.4 What are common indications for ventilating a patient during surgery? What are the potential adverse effects of using this technique?

3.5 Give six potential benefits of regional anaesthesia.

3.6 What factors predispose to regurgitation and aspiration of gastric contents? How can this be prevented?

3.7 What are the clinical signs that would suggest a patient is having an anaphylactic reaction? What would be your immediate management?

Chapter 4

Postanaesthesia care

The vast majority of patients recover from anaesthesia and surgery uneventfully, but a small and unpredictable number suffer complications. It is now accepted that all patients should be nursed by trained staff, in an area with appropriate facilities to deal with any of the problems that may arise while recovering from anaesthesia. Most patients will be nursed on a trolley capable of being tipped head-down. Patients who have undergone prolonged surgery or where a prolonged stay in recovery is expected may be nursed on their beds to minimize the number of transfers. Some patients who have undergone specialist surgery may be taken directly to a high dependency area, for example cardiac surgery patients.

The recovery unit

Each patient in the recovery unit should be cared for in an area equipped with:

- oxygen supply plus appropriate circuits for giving it;
- suction;
- ECG monitoring;
- pulse oximeter;
- non-invasive blood pressure monitor.

In addition, the following must be available immediately:

- *Airway equipment* Oral and nasal airways, a range of tracheal tubes, laryngoscopes, a bronchoscope, and the instruments to perform a cricothyroidotomy and tracheostomy.
- *Breathing and ventilation equipment* Self-inflating bag-valve-masks, a mechanical ventilator, and a chest drain set.
- *Circulation equipment* A defibrillator, drugs for cardiopulmonary resuscitation, a range of IV solutions, pressure infusers, and devices for IV access.
- *Drugs* For resuscitation and anaesthesia.
- *Monitoring equipment* Transducers and a monitor capable of displaying two or three pressure waveforms, an end-tidal CO_2 monitor, and a thermometer. This may be needed in patients who have undergone complex surgery with invasive monitoring that is continued in the immediate postoperative period, or occasionally those who require resuscitation.

Discharge of the patient

The anaesthetist's responsibility to the patient does not end with termination of the anaesthetic. Although care is handed over to the recovery staff (nurse or equivalent), the responsibility ultimately remains with the anaesthetist until the patient is discharged from the recovery area. If there are inadequate numbers of recovery staff to care for a newly admitted patient, the anaesthetist should adopt this role.

A patient who cannot maintain his/her own airway should never be left alone.

The length of time any patient spends in recovery will depend upon a variety of factors, including duration and type of surgery, anaesthetic technique, and the occurrence of any complications. Most units have a policy determining the minimum length of stay, (usually around 30 min), and agreed discharge criteria (Table 4.1).

Postoperative complications and their management

Hypoxaemia

This is the most important respiratory complication after anaesthesia and surgery. It may start at recovery, and in some patients persist for 3 days or more after surgery. The presence of cyanosis is very insensitive, and when detectable means the PaO_2 will be <8 kPa (55 mmHg), corresponding to a haemoglobin saturation of 85%. The advent of pulse oximetry has had a major impact on the prevention of hypoxaemia and should be used routinely in all patients. If hypoxaemia is severe, persistent, or when there is any doubt, arterial blood gas analysis should be performed. Hypoxaemia can be caused by a number of factors, either alone or in combination:

- alveolar hypoventilation;
- ventilation/perfusion mismatch within the lungs;
- diffusion hypoxia;
- pulmonary diffusion defects;
- a reduced inspired oxygen concentration.

Table 4.1 Minimum criteria for discharge from recovery area.

- Fully conscious and able to maintain own airway (although patient may still be 'sleepy')
- Adequate breathing
- Stable cardiovascular system, with minimal bleeding from the surgical site
- Adequate pain relief
- Warm

Alveolar hypoventilation

This is the most common cause of hypoxaemia after general anaesthesia. It is caused by a degree of respiratory depression leading to an insufficient flow of oxygen into the alveoli to replace that taken up by the blood. As a result alveolar $P\text{O}_2$ (PaO_2) and arterial $P\text{O}_2$ (PaO_2) fall. In most patients, increasing their inspired oxygen concentration will restore both. This is the rationale for giving all patients who have had a general anaesthetic oxygen therapy. Figure 4.1 shows the variation of PaO_2 with ventilation (minute volume). Note the effect of giving 30% oxygen to a patient whose ventilation is 2 L/min (normally 5 L/min): the PaO_2 rises from being barely adequate to supranormal. This is because 30% oxygen contains nearly one and a half times the amount of oxygen that is in air. If ventilation is further reduced, a point is eventually reached where there is only ventilation of the anatomical 'dead space', i.e. the volume of the airways that plays no part in gas exchange. If this occurs, irrespective of the inspired oxygen concentration, no oxygen reaches the alveoli and profound hypoxaemia will follow. Note that an increase in minute volume above normal only increases oxygenation minimally. This is because it does not alter the main determinant of alveolar oxygen tension, the inspired $P\text{O}_2$. Hypoventilation is always accompanied by hypercapnia, as there is an inverse relationship between alveolar ventilation and arterial carbon dioxide ($PaCO_2$) (Fig. 4.2).

Common causes of hypoventilation include:

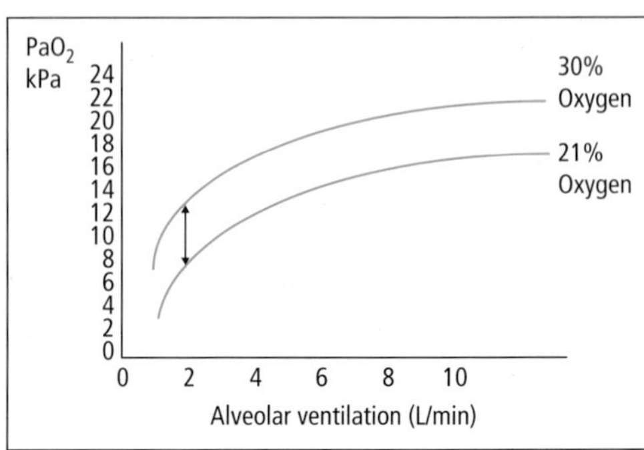

Fig. 4.1 Graph showing the relationship between PaO_2 and alveolar ventilation.

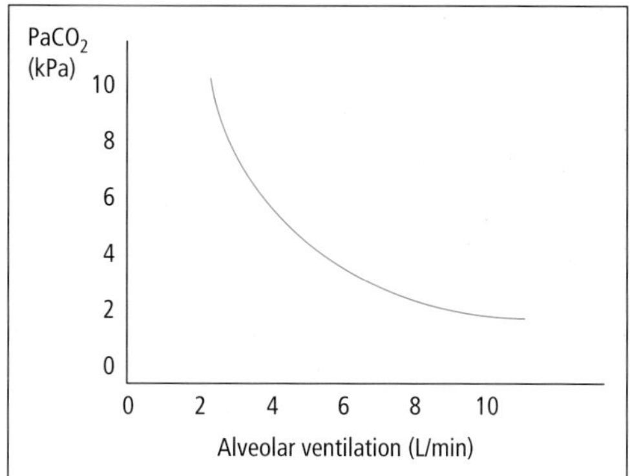

Fig.4.2 Graph showing the relationship between $PaCO_2$ and alveolar ventilation.

• *Obstruction of the airway* Most often due to the tongue. Consider vomit, blood, or swelling (e.g. post-thyroid surgery). Partial obstruction causes noisy breathing; in complete obstruction there is little noise despite vigorous efforts. There may be a characteristic 'see-saw' or paradoxical pattern of ventilation. A tracheal tug may be seen. The risk of obstruction can be reduced by recovering patients in the lateral position, particularly those recovering from surgery where there is a risk of bleeding into the airway (e.g. ENT surgery), or regurgitation (bowel obstruction or a history of reflux). If it is not possible to turn the patient (e.g. after a hip replacement), perform a chin lift or jaw thrust (see page 56). An oropharyngeal or nasopharyngeal airway may be required to help maintain the airway (see page 57).

> No patient should be handed to the care of the recovery nurse with noisy respiration of unknown cause.

• *Central respiratory depression* One of the effects of residual anaesthetic drugs is to depress the normal increase in ventilation seen in response to hypoxia and hypercarbia. Ventilation must be supported until the effects have worn off or been reversed. Opioid analgesics are a common cause of respiratory depression and, if severe, may require the specific antagonist naloxone to be given (see page 42).

• *Impaired mechanics of ventilation* Pain, particularly after upper abdominal or thoracic surgery, prevents coughing, leading to sputum retention and atelectasis. Provide adequate analgesia (consider central neural block). Residual neuromuscular blockade causes weakness and impaired ventilation. The patient will usually show signs of unsustained, jerky movements with rapid, shallow breathing, hypertension, and tachycardia. The diagnosis can be confirmed by using a peripheral nerve stimulator (see page 30). The patient should be given oxygen, reassured, sat upright to improve the efficiency of ventilation, and a (further) dose of neostigmine and an anticholinergic given.

• *Diaphragmatic splinting* Abdominal distension and obesity cause the diaphragm to be pushed into the thorax and increase the work of breathing. Sitting these patients up helps them greatly.

• *Cerebral haemorrhage or ischaemia* May cause direct damage to the respiratory centre or, more commonly, a deeply unconscious patient unable to maintain a patent airway.

• *Pneumothorax or haemothorax* Both will prevent ventilation of the underlying lung and will require the insertion of a chest drain.

• *Hypothermia* Reduces ventilation but, in the absence of any contributing factors, it is usually adequate for the body's needs.

Ventilation/perfusion mismatch within the lungs

Normally, alveolar ventilation (V) and perfusion with blood (Q) are well matched ($V/Q = 1$) and the haemoglobin in blood leaving the lungs is almost fully saturated with oxygen (97–98%). This is disturbed (ventilation/perfusion (V/Q) mismatch) during anaesthesia and the recovery period, with development of areas where:

• *Perfusion exceeds ventilation ($V/Q < 1$)*: this results in haemoglobin with a reduced oxygen content.

• *Ventilation exceeds perfusion ($V/Q > 1$)*: this can be considered wasted ventilation. Only a small additional volume of oxygen is taken up as the haemoglobin is already almost fully saturated.

In the most extreme situation, there is perfusion of areas of the lung but no ventilation ($V/Q = 0$). Blood leaving these areas remains 'venous' and is often referred to as 'shunted blood' (i.e. it is effectively shunted directly from the venous to arterial system). This is then mixed with oxygenated blood leaving ventilated areas of the lungs. The net result is:

- Blood perfusing alveoli ventilated with air has an oxygen content of approximately 20 mL/100 mL of blood.
- Blood perfusing unventilated alveoli remains venous, with an oxygen content of 15 mL/100 mL of blood.
- The final oxygen content of blood leaving the lungs will be dependent on the relative proportions of shunted blood and non-shunted blood.

> For an equivalent blood flow, areas of V/Q <1 decrease oxygen content more than areas of V/Q >1 can increase it, even if the inspired oxygen concentration is increased to 100%.

The aetiology of V/Q mismatch is multifactorial, but the following are recognized as being of importance:

- Mechanical ventilation reduces cardiac output. This reduces perfusion of non-dependent areas of the lungs, whilst maintaining ventilation. This is worst in the lateral position, when the upper lung is better ventilated and the lower lung better perfused.
- A reduced FRC. In supine, anaesthetized patients, particularly those over 50 years of age, the FRC falls below their closing capacity—the lung volume below which some airways close and distal alveoli are no longer ventilated. Eventually, areas of atelectasis develop, mainly in dependent areas of the lung that are perfused but not ventilated.
- Pain restricts breathing and coughing, leading to poor ventilation of the lung bases, sputum retention, basal atelectasis, and, ultimately, infection. The highest incidence of this is seen in the following circumstances:
  - smokers;
  - obesity;
  - pre-existing lung disease;
  - the elderly;
  - after upper gastrointestinal or thoracic surgery;
  - 3 days after surgery.

The effects of small areas of V/Q mismatch can be compensated for by increasing the inspired oxygen concentration. However, because of the disproportionate effect of areas where V/Q <1, once more than 30% of the pulmonary blood flow is passing through such areas, even breathing 100% oxygen will not eliminate hypoxaemia. The oxygen content of the blood leaving alveoli ventilated with 100% oxygen will only have increased by 1 mL/100 mL of blood over what was achieved when being ventilated with air (21 mL/100 mL of blood, Table 4.2). This is insufficient to offset the lack from the areas of low V/Q. Oxygen therapy is relatively ineffective when the cause of hypoxaemia is V/Q mismatch compared with when hypoventilation exists. Treatment should be aimed at optimizing ventilation of non-aerated alveoli. The simplest manoeuvre is to sit the patient upright in bed, which relieves upward pressure on the diaphragm, easing the work of breathing and so improving aeration of the lung bases. The next manoeuvre is to apply continuous positive airway pressure (CPAP) via a closely fitting facemask and a suitable circuit. This recruits alveoli but may be poorly tolerated by patients for periods of more than a few hours.

> Oxygen therapy is relatively ineffective at relieving hypoxaemia where the cause is V/Q mismatch compared with hypoventilation. Opening (recruiting) unventilated alveoli is likely to be more effective.

Table 4.2 Effect of alveolar oxygen concentration on oxygen content of blood.

	Alveolar oxygen concentration (%)	Haemoglobin saturation (%)	Oxygen content (mL/100 mL blood)
Alveoli containing air	21	97	20
Alveoli containing oxygen	100	100	21
Non-ventilated alveoli	Very low	75	15

Diffusion hypoxia

Nitrous oxide absorbed during anaesthesia has to be excreted during recovery. It is very insoluble in blood, and so rapidly diffuses down a concentration gradient into the alveoli, where it reduces the partial pressure of oxygen, making the patient hypoxaemic. This can be treated by giving oxygen via a facemask to increase the inspired oxygen concentration (see below).

Pulmonary diffusion defects

Any chronic condition causing thickening of the alveolar membrane, for example fibrosing alveolitis, impairs transfer of oxygen into the blood. In the recovery period it may also occur secondary to the development of pulmonary oedema following fluid overload or impaired left ventricular function. It should be treated by first administering oxygen to increase the partial pressure of oxygen in the alveoli and then by management of any underlying cause.

A reduced inspired oxygen concentration

As the inspired oxygen concentration is a prime determinant of the amount of oxygen in the alveoli, reducing this will lead to hypoxaemia. There are no circumstances where it is appropriate to administer less than 21% oxygen.

Management of hypoxaemia

All patients should be given oxygen in the immediate postoperative period to:

- counter the effects of diffusion hypoxia when nitrous oxide has been used;
- compensate for any hypoventilation;
- compensate for V/Q mismatch;
- meet the increased oxygen demand when shivering.

Patients who continue to hypoventilate, have persistent V/Q mismatch, are obese, anaemic, or have ischaemic heart disease will require additional oxygen for an extended period of time. The need for, and effectiveness of oxygen therapy is best determined either by arterial blood gas analysis or by using a pulse oximeter.

Devices used for delivery of oxygen

Variable-performance devices: masks or nasal cannulae

These are adequate for the majority of patients recovering from anaesthesia and surgery. The precise concentration of oxygen inspired by the patient is unknown as it is dependent upon the patient's respiratory pattern and the flow of oxygen used (usually 2–12L/min). The inspired gas consists of a mixture of:

- oxygen flowing into the mask;
- oxygen that has accumulated under the mask during the expiratory pause;
- alveolar gas from the previous breath which has collected under the mask;
- air entrained during peak inspiratory flow from the holes in the side of the mask and from leaks between the mask and face.

Examples of this type of device are Hudson and MC masks (Fig. 4.3). As a guide, they increase the

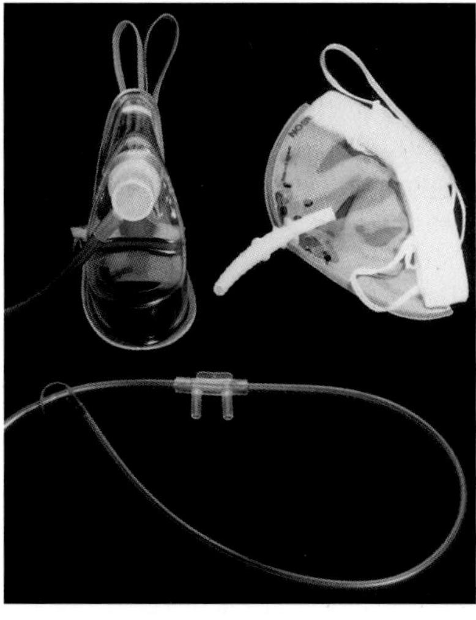

Fig. 4.3 Hudson mask (top left), MC mask (top right), and nasal catheters (bottom).

inspired oxygen concentration to 25–60% with oxygen flows of 2–12 L/min.

Patients unable to tolerate a facemask who can nose-breathe may find either a single foam-tipped catheter or double catheters, placed just inside the vestibule of the nose, more comfortable (see Fig. 4.3). Lower flows, 2–4 L/min, of oxygen are used, which increases the inspired oxygen concentration to 25–40%.

If higher inspired oxygen concentrations are needed in a spontaneously breathing patient, a Hudson mask with a reservoir bag can be used (see Fig. 4.4). A one-way valve diverts the oxygen flow into the reservoir during expiration. The contents of the reservoir, along with the high flow of oxygen (12–15 L/min), can almost meet the demand of peak inspiration gas flow, resulting in minimal entrainment of air, raising the inspired concentration to approximately 85%. An inspired oxygen concentration of 100% can only be achieved by using either an anaesthetic system with a close-fitting facemask or a self-inflating bag with reservoir and non-rebreathing valve, and an oxygen flow of 12–15 L/min.

Fixed-performance devices

These are used when it is important to deliver a precise concentration of oxygen, unaffected by the patient's ventilatory pattern, for example patients with COPD and CO_2 retention. These masks work on the principle of high airflow oxygen enrichment (HAFOE). Oxygen is fed into a Venturi that entrains a much greater but constant flow of air. The total flow into the mask may be as high as 45 L/min. The high gas flow has two effects: it meets the patient's peak inspiratory flow, reducing the volume of air drawn in around the mask, and flushes expiratory gas, reducing rebreathing. Masks deliver either a fixed concentration or have interchangeable Venturis to vary the oxygen concentration (Fig. 4.4).

The above systems all deliver dry gas to the patient, which may cause crusting or thickening of secretions and difficulty with clearance. For prolonged use, a HAFOE system should be used with a humidifier.

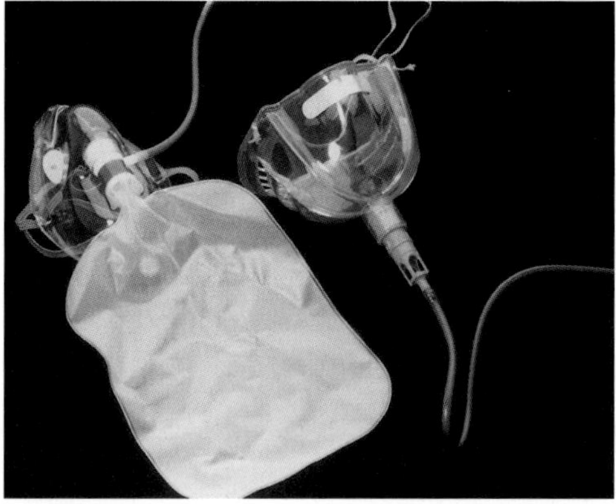

Fig. 4.4 Hudson mask with reservoir and high airflow oxygen enrichment (HAFOE; Venturi) mask.

Hypotension

This can be due to a variety of factors, alone or in combination:

- a reduction in circulating volume (preload);
- a reduced cardiac output (reduced myocardial contractility, valvular dysfunction, arrhythmias);
- vasodilatation (afterload);

These should be assessed and treated using a stepwise approach.

Step 1: assess the circulating volume (preload)

Hypovolaemia is the most common cause of hypotension after anaesthesia and surgery. Although intraoperative blood loss is usually obvious, continued bleeding, especially in the absence of surgical drains, may not be. Fluid loss may also occur as a result of tissue damage leading to oedema, or from evaporation during prolonged surgery on body cavities, for example the abdomen or thorax (see below). The diagnosis can be confirmed by finding:

- Reduced peripheral perfusion; cold clammy skin or delayed capillary refill (>2 s) in the absence of fear, pain, and hypothermia.
- Tachycardia; a pulse rate >100 beats/min of poor volume.
- Hypotension: initially, SBP may be reduced minimally but the DBP elevated as a result of compen-

satory vasoconstriction (narrow pulse pressure). The blood pressure must always be interpreted in conjunction with the other assessments.

- Inadequate urine output (<0.5 mL/kg/h), best measured hourly via a catheter and urometer.

Consider also the following as causes of reduced urine output:

  - a blocked catheter (blood clot or lubricant);
  - hypotension;
  - hypoxia;
  - renal damage intraoperatively (e.g. during aortic aneurysm surgery).

The most common cause of oliguria is hypovolaemia; anuria is usually due to a blocked catheter.

The extent to which these changes occur will depend primarily upon the degree of hypovolaemia. A tachycardia may not be seen in the patient taking beta-blockers, and a fit, young patient may lose up to 15% of their blood volume without detectable signs.

Management

- Ensure adequate oxygenation and ventilation.
- Give IV fluid, either crystalloid or colloid, using a pressure infusor if rapid resuscitation is required.
- Consider cross-matching blood if not already done.
- Stop any external haemorrhage with direct pressure.
- Get surgical assistance if internal haemorrhage suspected.
- In patients who have had a CVP line inserted, or had surgery close to or involving the pleura, consider a tension pneumothorax.

Monitoring of the patient's central venous pressure (CVP) may be indicated if cardiac function is in question. In the presence of significant hypovolaemia do not waste time inserting a CVP line for venous access alone. Fluids flow faster through short, wide bore tubes than long narrow ones. An arterial blood sample should be taken and analysed; a metabolic (lactic) acidosis is usually found after a period of poor tissue perfusion, and the trend of the patient's acid–base status is a useful indicator of therapeutic success.

Step 2: assess cardiac output

The most common causes of a reduction in cardiac output are left ventricular dysfunction due to ischaemic heart disease (or more rarely valvular heart disease) or an arrhythmia.

Left ventricular dysfunction

Having eliminated the factors above, the diagnosis should be considered on finding:

- poor peripheral circulation;
- tachycardia;
- tachypnoea;
- distended neck veins, raised jugular venous pressure (JVP);
- basal crepitations on auscultation of the lungs;
- wheeze with a productive cough;
- a triple rhythm on auscultation of the heart.

It is not uncommon to mistake this condition for hypovolaemia based on the first three findings. A chest X-ray may be diagnostic.

Management

- Sit the patient upright.
- Give 100% oxygen.
- Monitor the ECG, blood pressure, and peripheral oxygen saturation.

If the diagnosis is unclear, a fluid challenge (maximum 5 mL/kg) can be given and the response observed; an improvement in the circulatory status suggests hypovolaemia. Where there is no doubt about the diagnosis, fluids can be restricted initially and a diuretic (e.g. furosemide 20–40 mg) given IV. Trends in the CVP can be monitored as a guide to therapy. Patients with ventricular failure are best cared for in a critical care area. If there is acute myocardial infarction, contractility may only improve with the use of inotropes in conjunction with vasodilators, and this is best undertaken in a critical care area, usually a coronary care unit (CCU) or ICU. Unfortunately thrombolysis is contraindicated after surgery.

Arrhythmias

Disturbances of cardiac rhythm are a common cause of hypotension and occur more frequently in the presence of:

- hypoxaemia;
- hypovolaemia;
- hypercarbia;
- hypothermia;
- sepsis;
- pre-existing ischaemic heart disease;
- electrolyte abnormalities;
- acid–base disturbances;
- inotropes, antiarrhythmics, bronchodilators.

Correction of the underlying problem will result in spontaneous resolution of many arrhythmias. Specific intervention is required if there is a significant reduction in cardiac output and hypotension. The Resuscitation Council (UK) publishes guidelines that are regularly updated.

Tachycardias

Cardiac filling occurs during diastole, which is progressively shortened as the heart rate increases. The result is insufficient time for ventricular filling, leading to a reduced cardiac output and eventually a fall in blood pressure. If the contribution from atrial contraction is also lost (e.g. in atrial fibrillation) there is further compromise. As coronary artery flow is dependent on diastolic time (and DBP), myocardial ischaemia is more likely particularly in combination with hypotension.

- *Sinus tachycardia (>100 beats/min)* The most common arrhythmia after anaesthesia and surgery, usually as a result of pain or hypovolaemia. If there is associated pyrexia, it may be an early indication of sepsis. Treatment consists of oxygen, analgesia, and adequate fluid replacement. If the tachycardia persists, a small dose of a beta-blocker may be given IV whilst monitoring the ECG, providing there are no contraindications. Rarely, the development of an unexplained tachycardia after anaesthesia may be the first sign of MH.
- *Supraventricular tachycardia* The most common is atrial fibrillation usually secondary to ischaemic heart disease or the presence of sepsis. Treatment will depend on the rate and reduction in cardiac output:
  - heart rate ⩾150/min with critical perfusion will require cardioversion followed by IV amiodarone 300 mg over 1 h;
  - heart rate <150/min with good perfusion, consider amiodarone 300 mg IV over 1 h.

Bradycardias

Although a slow heart rate reduces myocardial oxygen demand and allows adequate time for ventricular filling, eventually the point is reached where end-diastolic volume is maximal, and further reductions in heart rate reduce cardiac output and hypotension ensues (remember cardiac output = heart rate × stroke volume).

- Sinus bradycardia (<60 beats/min) Usually the result of:
  - an inadequate dose of an anticholinergic (e.g. glycopyrrolate) given with neostigmine to reverse neuromuscular block;
  - excessive suction to clear pharyngeal or tracheal secretions;
  - traction on viscera during surgery;
  - excessive high spread of spinal or epidural anaesthesia;
  - the development of acute inferior MI;
  - excessive beta-blockade preoperatively or intraoperatively.

Treatment should consist of removing any provoking stimuli and administering oxygen. If hypotensive, atropine 0.5 mg IV should be given. If there is no response, consider an infusion of adrenaline, 2–10 μg/min or external pacing.

Rarely may be the result of a complete heart block which responds to external pacing until definitive treatment is arranged.

Step 3: assess for vasodilatation

This is common during spinal or epidural anaesthesia (see page 72), a typical example being after prostate surgery under spinal anaesthesia. As the legs are taken down from the lithotomy position, vasodilatation in the lower limbs is unmasked and, as the patient is moved to the recovery area, they become profoundly hypotensive. Hypotension secondary to regional anaesthesia is corrected by the administration of fluids (crystalloid, colloid), the use of vasopressors (e.g. ephedrine), or a combination of both. The combination of hypovolaemia and vasodilatation will cause profound hypotension. Oxygen should always be given.

Sometimes the cause of hypotension is multifactorial, as in septic shock where a patient may initially present with peripheral vasodilatation causing hypotension and tachycardia in the absence of blood loss. The patient may be pyrexial and, if the cardiac output is measured, it is usually found to be elevated. Gradually systemic sepsis ensues, causing reduced cardiac contractility, worsening hypotension, and poor perfusion, leading to an acidosis and arrhythmia, often atrial fibrillation. The diagnosis should be suspected in any patient who has had surgery associated with a septic focus, for example free infection in the peritoneal cavity or where there is infection in the genitourinary tract. This usually presents several hours after the patient has left the recovery area, often during the night following daytime surgery. The causative microorganism is often a Gram-negative bacterium. Patients developing septic shock require early diagnosis, invasive monitoring, and circulatory support in a critical care area. Antibiotic therapy should be guided by a microbiologist.

> When treating hypotension correct hypovolaemia before using inotropes.

Hypertension

This is most common in patients with pre-existing hypertension, but may be caused or exacerbated by:

- pain;
- hypoxaemia;
- hypercarbia;
- confusion or delirium;
- hypothermia.

Hypertension with coexisting tachycardia and in the presence of ischaemic heart disease is particularly dangerous as both increase myocardial work and oxygen consumption and may cause an acute MI. If the blood pressure remains elevated after correcting the above, a vasodilator or beta-blocker may be necessary. Senior help should be sought.

Postoperative nausea and vomiting (PONV)

This occurs in up to 80% of patients following anaesthesia and surgery. PONV is rarely fatal, but it is unpleasant and leaves patients feeling dissatisfied with the care they have received. Some patients would rather have the pain than the PONV. It may cause delayed discharge from hospital and thereby increase costs. For these reasons it is to be taken seriously, and measures should be employed to avoid it. A variety of factors have been identified which increase the incidence:

- Patient factors:
  - age and sex: more common in young women and children;
  - patients prone to travel sickness;
  - previous PONV;
  - being a non-smoker.
- Anaesthetic factors:
  - general anaesthesia compared with regional anaesthesia;
  - anaesthetic drugs: use of etomidate, nitrous oxide, opioid analgesics pre-, intra-, and postoperatively;
  - inhalational drugs compared with TIVA using propofol;
  - hypotension associated with epidural or spinal anaesthesia;
  - gastric dilatation, caused by manual ventilation with a bag and mask without a clear airway.
- Surgical factors:
  - site of surgery: abdominal, middle ear, gynaecological, ophthalmic, breast, or posterior cranial fossa.

Patients identified as being at risk of PONV should be given an antiemetic before emergence from anaesthesia because it is often easier to prevent vomiting than to stop it once it has started. Failure of treatment may be addressed in the recovery area by giving a second or third drug from the different classes of compounds below.

Drugs used to treat nausea and vomiting

Before resorting to the administration of drugs to treat nausea and vomiting, it is essential to make sure that the patient is not hypoxaemic or hypotensive. There are four main classes of drugs:

1 *5-HT3 (hydroxytryptamine) antagonists*. Ondansetron has proven efficacy in PONV and limited side-effects. It has both peripheral and central actions, blocking receptors in the gut (vagal afferents) and in the chemoreceptor trigger zone (CTZ). The dose in adults is 4–8 mg IV or orally 8 hourly.

2 *Antihistamines*. Cyclizine. Blocks H1 (histamine) and muscarinic receptors in the vomiting centre. Anticholinergic actions may cause a tachycardia when given IV, which can precipitate myocardial ischaemia in susceptible individuals and drowsiness. Avoid in patients with glaucoma. The dose in adults is 50 mg IM, up to 6 hourly.

3 *Dopamine antagonists*. Metoclopramide, domperidone. Block D2 (dopamine) receptors in the CTZ. Also have a prokinetic effect. Metoclopramide is relatively ineffective in PONV and may have extrapyramidal side-effects. Domperidone has fewer side-effects so is the preferred drug from this class. Phenothiazine derivatives such as prochlorperazine may block D2 and 5-HT receptors in the CTZ. The dose of metoclopramide is 10 mg IV, IM, or orally, 6 hourly; domperidone 10 mg orally 6 hourly.

4 *Anticholinergics*. Hyoscine. Inhibits stimulation of the vomiting centre by blocking muscarinic receptors in the vestibular system. Useful in patients who have had posterior cranial fossa surgery where PONV does not respond to the above drugs. Available as a transdermal patch. Causes a dry mouth and blurred vision.

Dexamethasone has been shown to be effective when given prophylactically and in combination with one or more of the above drugs. Its mechanism of action is not clear. The dose is 4–8 mg IV.

Most recovery units have a PONV pathway that may be printed onto a sticker and attached to the patient's drug chart for ease of use (Fig. 4.5).

Postoperative intravenous fluid therapy

A 70 kg man contains 45 L of water, of which 30 L are in the intracellular space and 15 L in the extracellular space. The latter is divided into the interstitial space (10 L) and the intravascular space (5 L). Daily water intake is approximately 2500 mL, comprising: 1500 mL orally, 750 mL in food, and 250 mL generated by the oxidation of carbohydrates. A similar volume is lost each day: 1500 mL as urine, 100 mL in faeces, and 900 mL as insensible losses (300 mL via the lungs, 600 mL via the skin). To maintain electrolyte balance, the following intake is required; sodium 1–1.5 mmol/kg, potassium 1 mmol/kg, and 0.1–0.2 mmol/kg each of calcium, magnesium, and phosphate. Inadequate water intake is sensed by osmo- and volume receptors that stimulate the release of antidiuretic hormone (ADH) and the sensation of thirst.

Minor surgery

All patients having an anaesthetic (and surgery) undergo a period of fasting pre- and intraoperatively, resulting in a water deficit. The loss comes from the total body water (ICF and ECF) which therefore has little effect on the intravascular volume. This is well tolerated when surgery is relatively minor and there is no significant blood loss. Providing that such patients resume oral intake 1–2 h postoperatively, they do not routinely need IV fluids in the perioperative period. The only exceptions to this are children and the elderly, who are very intolerant of even relatively minor degrees of dehydration, and those patients with a high risk of PONV where giving fluids may reduce the risk.

If surgery is prolonged, or a patient has failed to drink within 4–6 h of recovering from anaesthesia, usually as a result of PONV, IV fluid will be required. Providing that the volume of vomit is not excessive, only maintenance fluids are required. These are calculated at 1.5 mL/kg/h, but must take into account the accrued deficit.

For example, a 70 kg patient fasted from 0800 to 1400 h, who is still unable to take fluids by mouth at 1800 h, will require:

- 1.5 mL/kg/h to make up the deficit from 0800 to 1800 h = 1.5 × 70 (kg) × 10 (h) = 1000 mL;
- 1.5 mL/kg/h from 1800 to 0800 h the following morning = 1.5 × 70 × 14 = 1400 mL.

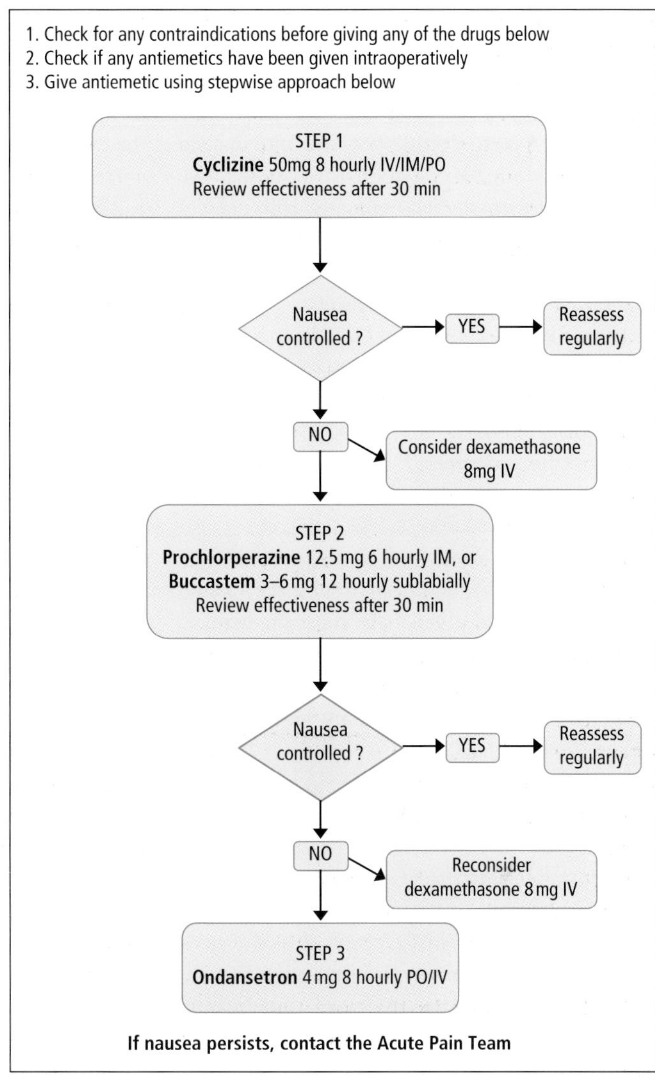

Fig. 4.5 Treatment pathway for postoperative nausea and vomiting (PONV).

The total IV fluid requirement = 2400 mL in the next 14 h if they are not able to resume oral intake.

An appropriate rate for the IV fluid would be:

- 1000 mL over the first 4 h;
- 1000 mL over the following 6 h;
- 500 mL over the last 4 h.

This should contain the daily requirement of Na^+ 1–1.5 mmol/kg and could be given either as:

2×1000 mL of 5% glucose and 500 mL of 0.9% (normal) saline; or

2×1000 mL of 4% glucose/0.18% saline, and 500 mL of 4% glucose/0.18% saline.

In practice most patients would probably be prescribed fluid at the rate of 1000 mL per 8 h either as 0.9% saline or as Hartmann's solution. Clearly this contains a greater amount of sodium than required, but this is easily excreted by the kidneys. Whatever regime is prescribed, the patient should be reviewed at 2200 h, and 0800 h the following morning to ensure that they are adequately hydrated (see below).

Major surgery

Postoperative fluid balance following major surgery is more complex. Assuming that appropriate volumes of water, electrolytes, and blood have been given during the operation, the postoperative fluid and electrolyte requirements will depend upon:

- the volume needed for maintenance, which will be increased if the patient is pyrexial;
- replacement of continuing losses from the gastrointestinal tract, for example via a nasogastric tube, fistulae, diarrhoea;
- losses into drains;
- any continued bleeding;
- rewarming of cold peripheries causing vasodilatation;
- the presence of an epidural for analgesia;
- the extent of tissue trauma or 'third space losses'.

Clearly every patient will have different requirements, and no single regime can cover all eventualities. The most important factor is clinical assessment and reassessment, along with appropriate monitoring.

Third space losses

The first and second spaces are the constituents of the ECF, namely the interstitial fluid space and the plasma. These are normal physiological compartments, and fluid shifts occur readily between them. A 'third space', related to and formed from the ECF, also exists and in non-pathological circumstances is usually referred to as the transcellular water, examples being CSF, urine, fluid within the gut, and fluids in the ducts of glands and serous cavities. Accumulation of third space fluid may also be pathological, examples being the swelling of tissues after surgical trauma or burns, ascites, pleural effusions, and fluid within the bowel lumen in a patient who has an ileus. In health, fluid intake replenishes the ECF, but in pathological conditions the interstitial and plasma fluid volumes become depleted in proportion to the volume of the third space losses. This has a proportionately greater effect on the plasma volume than if the losses were distributed from the total body water, for example in dehydration. The biggest problem for the clinician is that it is impossible to quantify such losses accurately; suffice it to say that the greater the degree of tissue damage from surgery or trauma, the greater the third space losses.

The patient who has undergone major surgery will require close monitoring to ensure that sufficient volumes of the correct fluid are given to replace what has been lost. These losses can be divided into two main groups; those that equate to ECF (blood, losses from the gastrointestinal tract, third space losses) and those that are mainly water (insensible losses). As seen above, the former will have a greater immediate effect as a significant part of the loss is from the plasma volume, and consequently will affect the perfusion and oxygenation of vital organs. This must be rectified rapidly. As already mentioned, water losses, unless excessive, have less of an effect on circulating volume and can be replaced more gradually.

In the first 24 h postoperatively no single regime can be provided, but the following must be taken into account when calculating and prescribing fluid therapy for each individual patient:

- maintenance fluids;
- 1.5 mL/kg/h water, increased by 10% for each °C if the patient is pyrexial;
- sodium, 1–1.5 mmol/kg;
- potassium 1.0 mmol/kg;
- replacement of measured gastrointestinal losses with an equal volume of 0.9% saline or Hartmann's solution;
- replacement of ongoing blood loss; aim for a haemoglobin concentration of 90 g/L;
  - <500 mL with either Hartmann's solution or 0.9% saline (up to three times the volume of blood lost as crystalloids are distributed throughout the ECF), or colloid, to the same volume as the blood loss;
  - >1000 mL may require transfusion with stored blood;
- replacement of ongoing losses into the third space;
- fluid required as a result of epidural induced vasodilatation.

Patients that have undergone major body cavity surgery may require large volumes of fluid postoperatively. In order to ensure that their demands are met, they must be regularly assessed, clinically, biochemically, and by the use of invasive monitoring, where appropriate.

Clinical assessment

- Thirst, dry mucous membranes; early reliable signs of dehydration.
- Cool peripheries, reduced skin turgor, tachycardia, oliguria, drowsiness; implies a significant fluid deficit.
- Hypotension, increased respiratory rate, coma; life threatening.
- Urine output, <0.5 mL/kg/h suggests significant hypovolaemia.

A review of the patient's observation charts looking at trends is often more useful than a 'snapshot' of their condition. Deterioration suggests that treatment is inadequate or that there are new or ongoing unidentified problems.

Biochemistry

- Raised haematocrit, urea, creatinine; support the diagnosis of dehydration.
- Metabolic acidosis; suggests hypovolaemia and hypoperfusion.

Monitoring

- CVP; normally 2–5 mmHg (3–8 cmH_2O), a low or negative CVP indicates fluid depletion. Trends are more useful, particularly the response to a fluid challenge; 250 mL of fluid are given rapidly and the change in CVP noted. In a hypovolaemic patient there will be a brief increase followed by a fall to the previous value. When the circulating volume is adequate there will be a small sustained rise. Overtransfusion will be seen as a high, sustained CVP.

On the second and subsequent days, the same basic principles are used. In addition:

- The fluid balance of the previous 24 h must be checked.
- Ensure that all sources of fluid loss are recorded.
- The patient's serum electrolytes must be checked to ensure adequate replacement and the fluid regime should be adjusted accordingly.
- The urine output for the previous 6 and 24 h should be noted; if decreasing, consider other causes of fluid loss, for example increasing pyrexia, development of an ileus.
- Magnesium and phosphate levels must be checked and replacements given if plasma concentrations are low.

The stress response

Following major surgery and trauma, matters are complicated further. Various neuroendocrine responses result in an increased secretion of a variety of hormones which have an effect on fluid balance. ADH secretion is maximal during surgery and may remain elevated for several days. The effect of this is to increase water absorption by the kidneys and reduce urine output. Aldosterone secretion is raised and, together with activation of the renin–angiotensin system, results in sodium and fluid retention and increased urinary excretion of potassium. Despite this retention of water and sodium, it is important that fluid input is not restricted in these patients, as the volume of the continued losses identified above is much more than the volume retained. Hence, in some patients, urine output may be as low as 0.5 mL/kg/h during the first two postoperative days without signifying organ hypoperfusion. This is particularly true after pulmonary and oesophageal surgery. It has been shown that in some cases reducing the volumes of fluid given and accepting a lower urine output results in fewer postoperative complications, as a result of less tissue oedema and fewer anastamotic breakdowns.

After 3–5 days, hormone levels return to normal, and this is followed by an increase in the volume of urine passed, which may be augmented as fluid sequestered to the pathological third space is reclaimed.

Postoperative analgesia

After injury, acute pain limits activity until healing has taken place. Modern surgical treatment restores function more rapidly, a process facilitated by the elimination of postoperative pain. A good example is the internal fixation of fractures, followed by potent analgesia allowing early mobilization. Ineffective treatment of postoperative pain not only delays this process, but also has other important consequences:

- Physical immobility:
  - reduced cough, sputum retention, and pneumonia;
  - muscle wasting, skin breakdown, and cardiovascular deconditioning;
  - thromboembolic disease—DVT and PE;
  - delayed bone and soft tissue healing.
- Psychological reaction:
  - reluctance to undergo further, necessary surgical procedures.
- Economic costs:
  - prolonged hospital stay, increased medical complications;
  - increased time away from normal occupations.
- Development of chronic pain syndromes.

Sometimes pain is a useful aid to diagnosis and must be recognized and acted upon, for example:

- pain due to a compartment syndrome;
- pain caused by dressings becoming too tight;
- pain of infection from cellulitis, peritonitis, or pneumonia;
- referred visceral pain in MI (arm or neck) or pancreatitis (to the back).

Any patient who complains of pain that unexpectedly increases in severity, changes in nature or site, or is of new onset should be examined to identify the cause rather than simply be prescribed analgesia.

Factors affecting the experience of pain

Pain and the patient's response to it are very variable and should be understood against the background of the individual's previous personal experiences and expectations rather than compared with the norm.

- Anxiety heightens the experience of pain. The preoperative visit by the anaesthetist plays a significant role in allaying anxiety by explaining what to expect postoperatively, what types of analgesia are available, and also by exploring patients' concerns with them.
- Patients who have a pre-existing chronic pain problem are vulnerable to suffering with additional acute pain. Their nervous systems can be considered to be sensitized to pain and will react more strongly to noxious stimuli. Bad previous pain experiences in hospital or anticipation of severe pain for another reason suggest that extra effort will be required to control the pain.
- Older patients tend to require lower doses of analgesics as a result of changes in drug distribution, metabolism, excretion, and coexisting disease. Prescribing should take these factors into account rather than using them as an excuse for inadequate analgesia. There is no difference between the intensity of pain suffered by the different sexes having the same operation.
- Upper abdominal and thoracic surgery cause the most severe pain of the longest duration, control of which is important because of the detrimental effects on ventilation. Pain following surgery on the body wall or periphery of limbs is less severe and for a shorter duration.

Management of postoperative pain

This can be divided into a number of steps:

- assessment of pain;
- analgesic drugs used;
- techniques of administration;
- difficult pain problems.

Assessment of acute pain

Regular measurement of pain means that it is less likely to be ignored and the efficacy of interventions can be assessed. There are a variety of methods of assessing pain; Table 4.3 shows a simple, practical system that is understood by patients and easily applied by staff. The numeric score is to facilitate recording and allows trends to be identified. Pain must be assessed with appropriate activity for the stage of recovery, for example 5 days after a hip joint replacement a patient would not be expected to have pain while lying in bed, but adequate

Table 4.3 A simple practical scoring system for acute pain.

Pain score	Staff view	Patient's view	Action
0	None	Insignificant or no pain	Consider reducing dose or changing to weaker analgesic, e.g. morphine to NSAID plus paracetamol
1	Mild	In pain, but expected and tolerable; no reason to seek (additional) treatment	Continue current therapy, review regularly
2	Moderate	Unpleasant situation; treatment desirable but not necessarily at the expense of severe treatment side-effects	Continue current therapy, consider additional regular simple analgesia, e.g. paracetamol and/or NSAID
3	Severe	Intolerable situation—will consider even unpleasant treatments to reduce pain	Increase dose of opioid, or start opioid; consider alternative technique, e.g. epidural

analgesia should allow mobilization with only mild to insignificant pain.

Analgesic drugs used postoperatively

The most commonly used drugs are opioids, NSAIDs, and local anaesthetics. Their sites of action are shown in Fig. 4.6.

Opioids

The pharmacology of opioid drugs and their side-effects are covered in Chapter 2. In the UK, morphine is widely used to control severe postoperative pain on surgical units and can be given by several routes (Table 4.4). One of the principal metabolites, morphine-6-glucuronide (M6G), has potent opioid effects and may accumulate and cause toxicity in patients with renal failure, particularly the elderly. Fentanyl and oxycodone have less active metabolites than morphine, and have faster onset of action, so may be more suitable for these patients.

For most painful clinical conditions there will be a blood level of opioid that provides useful analgesia, i.e. a reduction in pain level. The dose required to achieve this may vary enormously between patients as a result of differences in:

- pharmacodynamics: the effect of the drug on the body (via the receptors);
- pharmacokinetics: how the body distributes, metabolizes, and eliminates the drug;
- the nature of the stimulus;
- the psychological reaction to the situation.

The biggest step forward in the treatment of acute pain with opioids has been the recognition that individual requirements are very variable and the dose needs to be titrated for each patient:

- There is no minimum or maximum dose.
- Even with best practice some pain will remain.
- Minimum levels of monitoring and intervention are necessary for safe and effective use.
- Additional methods of analgesia should be considered if opioid requirements are high.

Overdose

Profound respiratory depression and coma due to opioids must be treated using the ABC principles described elsewhere (see Chapter 5). Having created a patent airway and supported ventilation using a bag-valve-mask with supplementary oxygen, the effects of the opioid can be pharmacologically reversed (antagonized) using naloxone. A dose of 0.4 mg is diluted to 5 mL with 0.9% saline and given in incremental doses of 1 mL IV (adult dosing). Analgesia will also be reversed, and careful thought must be given to continuing analgesia. HDU care is usually advisable in this situation.

Long-term complications of opioids

Adequate treatment of acute pain with opioids is not associated with dependency.

Non-steroidal anti-inflammatory drugs (NSAIDs)

The pharmacology of these drugs is covered in Chapter 2.

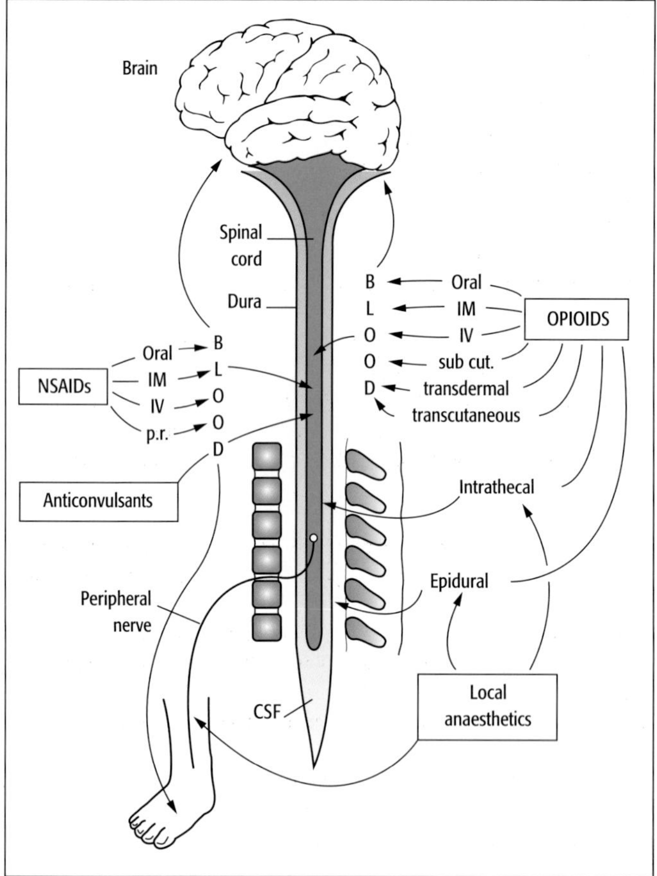

Fig. 4.6 Site of action of analgesic drugs.

Analgesic techniques used postoperatively

Patient-controlled analgesia (PCA)

- A microprocessor-controlled syringe pump capable of being programmed is used to deliver a predetermined dose of a drug IV.
- Activation is by the patient depressing a switch that is designed to prevent accidental triggering (hence 'patient-controlled').
- There may be a background, low-dose, continuous infusion.

To prevent the administration of an overdose:

- The maximum dose in any period and any background infusion is predetermined.
- After successful administration of a dose, a subsequent dose cannot be given for a preset period, the 'lockout period'.
- Typical settings for an adult using morphine delivered by a PCA device might be:
  - bolus dose: 1 mg;
  - lockout interval: 5 min.
- PCA devices record attempts made by the patient to access analgesia, allowing the dose to be adjusted to meet their requirements

Effective PCA requires:

- The patient to be briefed by the anaesthetist and/or nursing staff preoperatively and, if possible, be shown the device to be used.
- A loading dose of analgesic, usually IV before starting. Failure to do this will result in the patient being unable to get sufficient analgesia from the PCA device, and the system will fail.

Table 4.4 Morphine preparations.

Oral	Immediate release (IR) tablets or liquid • Absorption and effect within minutes • Usual adult dose 20 mg hourly prn • Less in elderly, more if opioid tolerant • Providing the gut is working, useful even after major surgery • Usually used for acute pain where the opioid requirement is unknown or changing rapidly Modified release (MR) tablets, capsules or granules • Dose released over either 12 or 24 h • Avoids frequent dosing with IR preparations • Useful when opioid requirement is prolonged and also for gradually weaning down the dose at the end of treatment The two formulations are usually used together to provide a steady background level of analgesia (MR) with additional breakthrough doses (IR) as required *It is important that everybody understands the difference between MR and IR forms of morphine*
Intravenous	Morphine 10 or 20 mg diluted to 1 mg/mL with 0.9% sodium chloride can be given: • In increments initially of 1–3 mg at 3 min intervals; effective dose may range from 1 to 50 mg or more (the latter in opioid-tolerant patients) • Via a PCA device (see text) • As a continuous infusion. Useful where patient cooperation is limited, e.g. in elderly patients or ICUs. Problems occur in predicting the correct infusion rate, given the variability of dose requirement between patients Very close supervision is required to avoid underinfusion (pain) or overinfusion (toxicity) This method can be used to replace high doses of oral opioids during the perioperative period *The IV dose of morphine is about one-third of the oral dose*
Intramuscular	• A predetermined dose (e.g. morphine 10 mg) at fixed minimum intervals, e.g. hourly • Delayed and variable rate of effect • Precise titration is difficult with repeated cycles of pain and relief • Does not require complex equipment or a cooperative patient • Although widely available, gradually being replaced by the above.

• A dedicated IV cannula or non-return valve on an IV infusion to prevent accumulation of the drug and failure of analgesia.

Observation and recording of the patient's pain score, sedation score, and respiratory rate is essential to ensure success. Any patient with a respiratory rate <8 breaths/min and a sedation score of 2 or 3 requires immediate intervention:

• Stop the PCA.
• Give oxygen via a mask.
• Call for assistance.
• Consider giving naloxone (see above).
• If the patient is apnoeic, commence ventilation using a self-inflating bag-valve-mask device.

Advantages of PCA

• Greater flexibility; analgesia matched to the patient's perception of the pain.
• Reduced workload for the nursing staff.
• Elimination of painful IM injections.
• IV administration with greater certainty of adequate plasma levels.

Disadvantages

• Equipment is expensive to purchase and maintain.
• Requires patient comprehension of the system.
• Patient must be physically able to trigger the device.
• The elderly are often reluctant to use a PCA device.
• The potential for overdose if the device is incorrectly programmed.

As pain subsides, the PCA can be discontinued, and oral analgesics can be used. The first dose should be

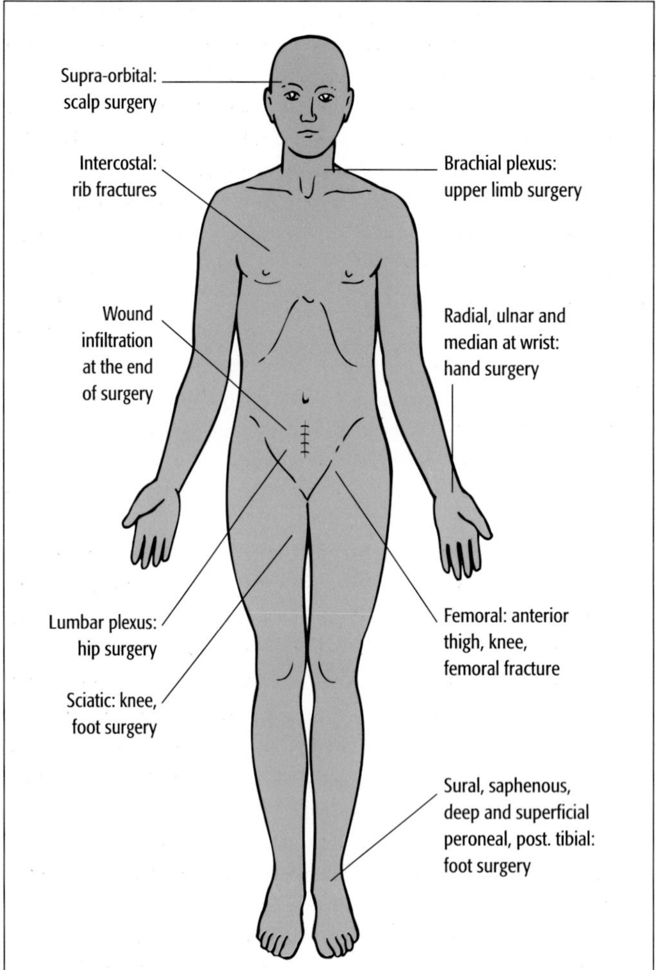

Fig. 4.7 Some commonly used nerve blocks.

given 1 h prior to discontinuing PCA, to ensure continuity of analgesia.

Regional analgesic techniques (Fig. 4.7)

- *Peripheral nerve blocks* Used mainly for pain relief after upper or lower limb surgery. A single injection of local anaesthetic, usually bupivacaine, results in 6–12 h of pain relief. An infusion of local anaesthetic via a catheter inserted close to the nerve may enable the block to be continued for several days. An alternative and effective form of analgesia must be prescribed for when the local anaesthetic is discontinued to prevent the patient being in severe pain.
- *Epidural analgesia (see also page 69)* Infusions of a local anaesthetic into the epidural space, either alone or in combination with opioids, act on the transiting nerve roots and the dorsal horn of the spinal cord, respectively, to provide dramatic relief of postoperative pain. It is essential that patients who are offered an epidural receive an explanation by the anaesthetist at the preoperative visit of what to expect postoperatively, in particular altered sensation, weakness of the lower limbs, and the potential need for a urinary catheter. The epidural is often sited preoperatively and used intraoperatively as part of the anaesthetic technique. For upper abdominal surgery an epidural in the mid-thoracic

region (T6/7) is used, while a hip operation would need a lumbar epidural (L1/2).

Different combinations of local anaesthetic and opioid infusion have been used successfully. Ideally, the concentration of local anaesthetic should selectively block sensory nerves, with relative sparing of motor nerves. The choice and dose of opioid should be such that the drug passes through the dura into the CSF in sufficient quantities to block the opioid receptors in the spinal cord but not spread cranially to cause respiratory depression. For example:

- bupivacaine 0.125% plus fentanyl 2–4 μg/mL.

Epidural infusions can be used to maintain analgesia for several days. Opioid side-effects are less common and less severe than when given systemically as the dose is much less.

Points to note

- The infusion rate and the site of the catheter determine the spread of the solution. In the thoracic epidural space a starting infusion rate might be 4 mL/h; in the lumbar space commence at 8 mL/h.
- The efficacy of the infusion must be monitored in a similar manner as for PCA.
- If analgesia is inadequate, a 'top-up' of 3–4 mL of solution may be necessary.
- Observations of the patient's vital signs should then be made on a regular basis according to local protocol.
- In patients over the age of 60 years, the concentration of opioid is often halved.

Management of complications during postoperative epidural analgesia

This will depend upon whether local anaesthetics alone or in combination with opioids have been used. The complications arising as a result of the use of local anaesthetics are the same as when they are used intraoperatively, and are covered in Chapter 3.

- *Hypotension* Sympathetic block causes vasodilatation and increased venous pooling. Treat acutely with IV fluid and vasopressors (e.g. ephedrine according to local policy). Prevented by ensuring the patient has an adequate fluid regimen prescribed. Patients with additional fluid losses, for example haemorrhage, are particularly vulnerable to severe hypotension. Check the extent of the block; if extensive, reduce the rate of infusion.
- *Respiratory depression* Caused by opioid reaching the respiratory centre in the medulla. Highly lipid-soluble opioids (diamorphine, fentanyl) are rapidly taken up by the spinal cord, limiting their spread and systemic absorption, and respiratory depression tends to occur early; less soluble opioids (morphine) are taken up slowly, and respiratory depression tends to occur later. A high infusion rate of either drug may also lead to respiratory depression. This can be prevented by regular assessment and recording of vital signs. Treat by supporting ventilation if necessary; stop the epidural infusion; give naloxone according to the severity; seek expert help.
- *Sedation* Due to opioid reaching the brain either directly via the CSF or after absorption into the systemic circulation via the epidural veins. It may also be secondary to hypotension and cerebral hypoxaemia. Prevent by regular assessment and recording of vital signs. Treat by stopping the infusion; if unresponsive or the level of sedation progresses, give naloxone in 0.1 mg increments IV; seek expert help.
- *Pruritus* Can be severe and frequently localized to the nose; may respond to antihistamines, atropine, or naloxone.
- *Retention of urine* May be due to the effect of the opioid on bladder sphincter control or the local anaesthetic removing the sensation of a full bladder. More common in males, particularly if there are already symptoms of prostatism. Prevented by routine monitoring of urine output in all postoperative patients. May require short-term catheterization.
- *Numbness and weakness of the legs* Usually due to excessive rates of infusion or a too-high concentration of local anaesthetic. May lead to pressure ulcers on the patient's heels or sacrum due to lack of movement, or falls whilst mobilizing. Prevented by regular observation of effects of epidural and correct adjustment of infusion rate.
- *Vertebral canal haematoma* Can occur as a result of trauma by the needle or catheter insertion. The risk is greater in patients on warfarin, heparin,

NSAIDs, and other antiplatelet drugs, those with a coagulopathy or when severely haemodiluted. Rare, but consider if profound motor and sensory block is far greater than anticipated.

• *Infection* Introduced via the catheter. May cause the formation of an epidural abscess and compromise of the spinal cord. Patients complain typically of increasing back pain, but this may be delayed for several weeks so that the connection to the surgery and epidural may be missed.

If there is any doubt about spinal cord function, the epidural infusion should be stopped and a magnetic resonance imaging (MRI) scan considered. Damage to nerves or the spinal cord during insertion of the needle and systemic toxicity of the local anaesthetic are both unusual complications.

Intrathecal (spinal) analgesia

Spinal anaesthesia is of insufficient duration to provide postoperative pain relief. However, if a small dose of opioid, for example morphine 0.1–0.25 mg, is injected along with the local anaesthetic, this may provide up to 24 h of analgesia. Complications are the same as those due to opioids given epidurally, and are managed in the same way.

Other techniques

Entonox is a mixture of nitrous oxide (50%) and oxygen (50%). It is a weak analgesic with sedative properties. Useful for short-term analgesia for painful procedures, for example change of dressings. It should be avoided in patients with a pneumothorax because the nitrous oxide may diffuse into the gas-filled space, increasing the volume.

Combining analgesic techniques

Examples of good practice are:

• bupivacaine and fentanyl in an epidural infusion;

• IV PCA morphine and IV paracoxib in the early postoperative period when nil by mouth;

• oral morphine immediate release (IR) tablets and paracetamol prescribed to be given as a spinal wears off.

Difficult pain problems

Patients who show evidence of regular opioid use preoperatively, for example drug addicts, cancer and chronic pain patients, and those patients with a previous bad pain experience, may pose a particular problem postoperatively. They are best managed if they are identified at the preoperative assessment and a team approach is used that will include:

• Liaison with the Acute Pain Team to inform them of the patient's admission.

• Discussion with the anaesthetist, and surgical and nursing staff to plan perioperative care, to:
  ○ ensure any current opioid medication is continued on admission to prevent withdrawal;
  ○ understand that much larger doses of opioids than normal may be required;
  ○ explain that toxicity from high doses of opioid is very unlikely;
  ○ reassure that addiction is not a concern.

• Discussion with the patient to explain:
  ○ types and effectiveness of analgesic regimes available postoperatively;
  ○ that analgesia may not be 100% effective;
  ○ that long-term continuation may be necessary;
  ○ potential side-effects, especially if regional analgesia planned.

• Plan regular reviews during postoperative period.

• Coordination of care.

Further reading

Bay I, Nunn JF, Prys Roberts C. Factors affecting arterial PO_2 during recovery from general anaesthesia. *British Journal of Anaesthesia* 1968; **40**: 398–407.

Gan TJ, Meyer T, Apfel CC *et al.*, and Department of Anesthesiology, Duke University Medical Center. Consensus guidelines for managing postoperative nausea and vomiting. *Anesthesia and Analgesia* 2003; **97**: 62–71.

Shelly MP, Eltringham RJ. Rational fluid therapy during surgery. *British Journal of Hospital Medicine* 1988; **39**: 506–17.

Thomson AJ, Webb DJ, Maxwell SRJ, Grant IS. Oxygen therapy in acute medical care. *British Medical Journal* 2002; **324**: 1406–7.

West JB. *Respiratory physiology: the essentials*, 6th edn. Baltimore: Williams and Wilkins, 1999.

Useful websites

http://www.aagbi.org/publications/guidelines/docs/postanaes02.pdf
[Immediate postanaesthetic recovery. The Association of Anaesthetists of Great Britain & Ireland. September 2002.]

http://oac.med.jhmi.edu/res_phys/
[The Johns Hopkins School of Medicine interactive respiratory physiology website.]

http://www.resus.org.uk/pages/periarst.pdf
[Current Resuscitation Council UK guidelines on peri-arrest arrhythmias.]

http://www.jr2.ox.ac.uk/bandolier/booth/painpag/
[The Oxford Pain site. Brilliant for the latest evidence-based information on all aspects of acute pain.]

http://www.jr2.ox.ac.uk/bandolier/Extraforbando/APain.pdf
[Acute Pain. Bandolier extra. Evidence-based healthcare. February 2003.]

http://www.rcoa.ac.uk/docs/ARB-section3.pdf
[Audit topics and useful information about postoperative care from The Royal College of Anaesthetists.]

http://www.asahq.org/publicationsAndServices/postanes.pdf
[Practice Guidelines for Postanesthetic Care. A Report by the American Society of Anesthesiologists Task Force on Postanesthetic Care.]

All websites last accessed April 2008.

Self-assessment

4.1 List the three main causes of hypoxaemia immediately postoperatively and give examples of a cause of each. What devices could be used to treat this problem and what concentration of oxygen will each deliver?

4.2 What are the three main causes of hypotension in the immediate postoperative period? What would be your immediate management?

4.3 Calculate the fluid requirement for the next 24-hours in a 60-year-old man at 0900, who had a laparotomy the previous afternoon. He weighs 80 kg and is apyrexial, his BP is 95/65 mmHg, pulse rate 110/min and he is complaining of feeling thirsty. In the last 12 hours he has passed 340 ml urine and lost 400 ml via a nasogastric tube. His serum sodium is 137 mmol/l, potassium 3.2 mmol/l and Hb 72 g/l.

4.4 Describe how a patient-controlled analgesia (PCA) device works. What are the advantages and disadvantages of such a device?

4.5 What are the five most common complications resulting from the use of epidural opiates for postoperative analgesia and how are they treated?

Chapter 5

Recognition and management of the acutely ill patient on the ward

With the exception of a few, often fatal, conditions such as massive PE, most critical illness does not occur instantly. The signs of a patient's physiological deterioration often develop gradually, evolving over many hours, and reflect failing cardiovascular, respiratory, renal, and neurological systems. Once a patient has developed organ failure that requires ICU admission, the risk of further complications and in-hospital death rises significantly. Some patients deteriorate to the point of cardiac arrest before the severity of their condition is recognized. The average in-hospital survival rate once cardiac arrest has occurred is approximately 17%, but for many patients on general wards the survival rate is much lower. Optimal management of the patient's primary pathology, early detection and appropriate management of any deterioration, and timely referral to ICU may help reduce this mortality.

Detecting acute illness

Numerous studies have identified that abnormalities in heart rate, blood pressure, respiratory rate, and conscious level signify impending critical events. Consequently, regular assessment of vital signs is fundamental to the early detection of the onset and progression of acute illness. NICE has recommended that adult patients admitted to hospital, or in whom a clinical decision to admit has been made, should have vital signs recorded at the time of their admission or initial assessment. These observations should be repeated at least every 12 h and more frequently if abnormal physiology is detected. Following this guidance should provide reliable and early detection of clinical deterioration, thereby allowing earlier interventions.

Track and trigger systems

Following the publication of the Department of Health's document 'Comprehensive Critical Care' in 2000, the use of 'track and trigger' systems to assist ward staff to identify 'at risk' or critically ill patients has become increasingly popular. These systems can be categorized into:

- Single- and multiple-parameter systems. In these systems 'normal limits' are set for a number of bedside observations, for example respiratory rate 10–30 breaths/min. The system is triggered if one or more of the parameters falls outside the 'normal range'.
- Aggregate weighted scoring systems. In these systems, each bedside observation is given a score, usually 0–3 based upon their degree of abnormality, with zero representing normality. The sum of the individual scores triggers further action, which can range from more frequent observations to obtaining senior medical help. An example of this type of system used in the UK is the Modified Early Warning Scoring System (MEWSS) (Table 5.1).

In both systems, another subjective category may be added 'any patient about whom there are

Table 5.1 The Modified Early Warning Scoring System.

Score	**3**	**2**	**1**	**0**	**1**	**2**	**3**
HR	<40	40–50	51–100	101–110	111–129	≥130	
BP	>45%↓	30%↓	15%↓	Normal*	15%↑	30%↑	>45%↑
RR	<8	9–14	15–20	21–29	≥30		
Temperature		<35.0°C		35.0–38.4°C		≥38.5°C	
CNS**				A	V	P	U
Urine	Nil	<0.5 mL/kg/h	<1 mL/kg/h		>1.5 mL/kg/h		

HR, heart rate; BP, blood pressure; RR, respiratory rate; CNS, central nervous system.

*Normal for patient.

**Assessment of conscious level: A, alert; V, responsive to verbal stimulus; P, responsive to painful stimulus; U, unresponsive.

Adapted from Stenhouse C, Coates S *et al*. Prospective evaluation of a modified Early Warning Score to aid earlier detection of patients developing critical illness on a surgical ward. *British Journal of Anaesthesia* 2000; **84**: 663P.

serious concerns', irrespective of the objective score. When such a concern is voiced by an experienced nurse, it should not be ignored!

Receiving a call

If called to assess an acutely ill patient you may not have seen him/her previously and may have no prior knowledge of his/her medical history. Therefore, when answering a call to assess a sick patient it is very helpful to obtain some information over the phone so that you can be thinking about possible causes and treatment as you make your way to the ward. An experienced referrer may provide a concise summary of the patient's recent history and current condition. However, if no information is volunteered you should ask a few pertinent questions:

- How old is the patient?
- When were they admitted to hospital?
- What is their working diagnosis?
- Are they conscious and, if so, what are they complaining of?
- How quickly have they deteriorated?
- What are their latest vital signs?
- Do they have a DNaR (do not attempt resuscitation) order?

The principles of assessment

When assessing and managing any acutely ill patient, irrespective of the severity of their condition, the primary aim must be to make the patient safe rather than to determine a precise diagnosis. Many clinical crises can be managed initially by prompt recognition and correction of a modest number of common abnormalities using simple therapies (e.g. oxygen and fluids). It is logical for all members of the healthcare team to use the same systematic approach to assess and treat the 'at risk' or acutely ill patient incorporating the following:

- Immediate assessment and treatment using an 'ABCDE' approach
- Start simple bedside monitoring
- A full assessment of the patient using all available information
- Decision making
- A definitive management or care plan
- Good record keeping.

Key points:

1 The aim of initial interventions is to keep the patient alive and produce some clinical improvement, such that definitive treatment may be initiated.
2 Always correct life-threatening abnormalities before moving on to the next stage of the assessment.
3 Resuscitation measures (oxygen, fluids, etc) often take a few minutes to have an effect.
4 Call for help early. At every stage of the patient assessment, consider ***"Do I need help?"***

Once the patient is made safe, undertake a full initial assessment and re-assess regularly to identify the impact of treatment and to detect patient deterioration. Don't try to do everything yourself; use all members of the multidisciplinary team, they are there to help you. To do this you must communicate effectively with everyone, staff, patients, and relatives.

There may be several interventions happening at the same time, particularly if the patient is in a periarrest situation; always ensure your own safety and that of the patient:

- Take note of environmental hazards—electricity, fluid spillage, etc.
- Dispose of needles and other sharps into 'sharps bins'.

Protective aprons, gloves, and masks will reduce the risk of contamination from secretions, blood, etc.

Staff hygiene has an important impact on patient outcome, therefore despite all the pressures:

- Always wash hands before and after patient contact.
- Use aseptic techniques for invasive procedures.

Initial approach to the patient

Ask the patient a simple question, such as 'How are you?' A normal verbal response immediately informs you that the patient:

- has a patent airway;
- is breathing;
- has brain perfusion with oxygenated blood.

If the patient can only speak in short sentences, suspect severe respiratory distress. Failure to respond to the question is likely to suggest serious illness, and you should immediately assess the patient for signs of life whilst keeping the airway open. If the patient has no signs of life, follow the current guidelines for in-hospital resuscitation (see page 117).

The next step is to commence an ABCDE assessment of the patient. While you are doing this, ask an assistant to attach the following as soon as is safely possible:

- Pulse oximeter.
- ECG monitor.
- Non-invasive blood pressure monitor.

The ABCDE system

A is for AIRWAY
B is for BREATHING
C is for CIRCULATION
D is for DISABILITY (i.e. CNS function)
E is for EXPOSURE (permitting full patient examination).

The assessment and consequent actions are prioritized in this order because, generally, airway obstruction kills faster than breathing disorders, which in turn kill faster than blood loss or cardiac dysfunction. Each part of the assessment system follows a similar pattern; the identification of potentially life-threatening emergencies and treatment of them simultaneously.

Most abnormalities will be detected using simple clinical examination techniques based on a look–feel–listen approach. The order of the various components of the look–feel–listen approach will vary depending on the body system being examined.

Assessing the state of the airway (A)

The aim is to identify and treat airway obstruction. Always treat airway obstruction as a medical emergency and obtain expert help immediately. Untreated, it leads to a lowered PaO_2, risks hypoxic damage to tissues (e.g. brain, kidneys, heart), and will eventually cause cardiac arrest and death. In a critically ill patient, airway obstruction is frequently due to a depressed conscious level, but there are many other causes (Table 5.2). The converse is also true.

Look for the signs of airway obstruction:

- Paradoxical chest and abdominal movements ('see-saw' respirations).
- Use of the accessory muscles of respiration (e.g. sternomastoid and muscles of the neck, back, and shoulder girdle).
- NOTE: central cyanosis is a late sign of airway obstruction.

Feel for the presence of air movement at the mouth:

- Place your face or hand immediately in front of the patient's mouth.

Table 5.2 Causes of airway obstruction.

Upper airway obstruction	Lower airway obstruction
• Depressed conscious level	• Secretions
• Secretions	• Blood
• Foreign body	• Vomit or gastric fluid
• Blood	• Laryngeal spasm
• Vomit or gastric fluid	• Laryngeal oedema
• Soft tissue swelling:	• Surgery
• trauma	• infection
• surgery	• burns
• inflammation	• anaphylaxis
• burns	• Tracheal or bronchial obstruction
• anaphylaxis	• secretions
• infection	• vomit
• pulmonary oedema	• bronchospasm

Table 5.3 The characteristics of airway noises assist in localizing the level of airway obstruction.

Sound	Cause
Gurgling	Liquid in the mouth or upper airway
Snoring	Partial obstruction of the pharynx, usually by the tongue
Crowing	Laryngeal spasm
Inspiratory stridor	Obstruction above or at the level of the larynx
Expiratory wheeze	Airway collapse during expiration (e.g. asthma)
Rattling	Secretions in the airways

Listen for the signs of airway obstruction:

- In complete upper airway obstruction, there are no breath sounds at the mouth or nose.
- In partial airway obstruction, air entry is diminished and often noisy.
- Certain noises assist in localizing the level of the obstruction (Table 5.3).

Noisy breathing ALWAYS indicates obstruction, silence may mean apnoea.

If there are signs of obstruction, call for expert help immediately and move rapidly to using simple methods of airway clearance, for example head tilt and chin lift (Figs 3.3 and 3.4), airways suction, and insertion of an oropharyngeal or nasopharyngeal airway (see Chapter 3). When these measures fail, tracheal intubation may be required, but should only be attempted by experienced staff. In most situations, intubation will require the use of hypnotic and neuromuscular blocking drugs.

Once an airway has been created, give oxygen at high concentration using a mask with an oxygen reservoir (Fig. 4.4), and move on rapidly to assess breathing.

Assessing breathing (B)

The aim is to assess adequacy of breathing. If untreated, inadequate breathing will lead to hypoxaemia and will also cause hypercapnia (see Figs 4.1 and 4.2) that can eventually lead to unconsciousness. There are many causes of disordered or inadequate breathing (see Table 5.4).

Look for the signs of abnormal breathing:

- Use of the accessory muscles of respiration, abdominal breathing, sweating, central cyanosis.
- Altered respiratory rate; normal is between 12 and 20 breaths/min. Higher rates, or those that are rising, are markers of illness and should be

Primary lung dysfunction	Secondary causes

• Pneumonia
• Acute asthma
• Acute exacerbation of COPD
• Emphysema
• Pulmonary fibrosis
• Pneumothorax/haemothorax
• Pulmonary contusion
	• Exhaustion
	• ARDS
	• Acute heart failure
	• Pulmonary embolism
	• Airway obstruction
	• Neuromuscular problems
	  • myopathies
	  • neuropathies
	  • Guillain–Barré syndrome
	• Myasthenia gravis
	• Spinal cord injury
	• CNS depression
	  • drugs
	  • head injury
	  • meningitis/encephalitis
	  • cerebral haemorrhage
	  • cerebral tumour
	  • cerebral hypoxia
	• Diaphragmatic splinting
	  • morbidly obese patients
	  • abdominal pain
	  • abdominal distension

Table 5.4 Causes of breathing problems.

regarded as a warning that the patient may suddenly deteriorate. Very low rates suggest a CNS problem.

Observe and assess the:

• Depth of each breath.

• Pattern (rhythm) of breathing.

• Equality of movement of the two sides of the chest.

Look for:

• Chest deformity, as this may impair the ability to breathe normally.

• Raised JVP (may signify acute severe asthma or a tension pneumothorax).

• Chest drains—assess if they are patent and draining.

• Abdominal distension, as this exacerbate respiratory distress by limiting diaphragmatic movement.

Feel the chest for:

• The position of the trachea in the suprasternal notch. Deviation to one side indicates mediastinal shift (e.g. pneumothorax, lung fibrosis, or pleural fluid).

• Surgical emphysema or crepitus (assume that this indicates a pneumothorax until proven otherwise).

• Percuss the chest; hyper-resonance suggests a pneumothorax; dullness suggests consolidation or pleural fluid.

Listen for the signs of respiratory disease:

• The patient's breath sounds a short distance from his/her face. Rattling or gurgling airway noises indicate the presence of airway secretions, usually due to the inability of the patient to cough sufficiently or to take a deep breath. Stridor or wheeze suggests partial, but significant, airway obstruction.

• Auscultate the chest: assess the quality of the breath sounds. Bronchial breathing indicates lung consolidation; absent or reduced sounds suggest the presence of a pneumothorax or pleural fluid.

If the patient's breathing is dangerously inadequate, they are apnoeic, or they have been intubated, high concentration oxygen must be given using a bag-valve-mask system (Fig. 5.1) whilst calling urgently for expert help. The addition of a

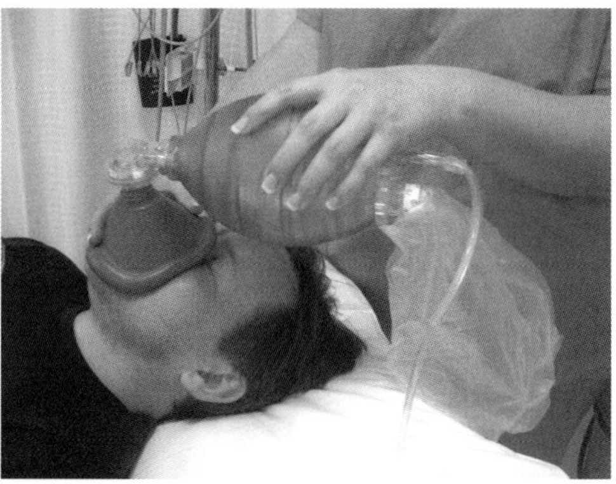

Figure 5.1 Ventilation with a self-inflating bag-valve-mask. There is an oxygen supply and reservoir attached to the bag to maximize the inspired oxygen concentration.

reservoir allows oxygen concentrations close to 100% to be given. As soon as possible, record their $Sp{O_2}$ (normally 97–99%) and inspired oxygen concentration (%). If possible treat any obvious underlying cause, for example acute severe asthma, pulmonary oedema, or tension pneumothorax.

In most patients, the target $Sp{O_2}$ should be above 95%. In patients suffering from COPD and breathing spontaneously, high concentrations of oxygen may have disadvantages and limiting the $Fi{O_2}$ may be warranted. Nevertheless, this latter group of patients remains at risk of end-organ damage, cardiac arrest, or death if their blood oxygen tensions are allowed to fall too low. In this group, aim for a target $Sp{O_2}$ of 90%.

If skilled help is available, send arterial blood for blood gas analysis. Alternatively this may be done at the end of 'C'. This will provide the information on the patient's:

- Oxygenation, PaO_2: as a 'rule of thumb' a difference between the $Pa{O_2}$ and inspired oxygen concentration (in kPa ≈ %) of more than 10 kPa implies a defect in oxygen uptake.
- Ventilation, $PaCO_2$: hypercapnia (increased $PaCO_2$) is the result of inadequate alveolar ventilation; hypocapnia, excessive ventilation.
- Metabolism, pH, base excess: sick patients usually have a metabolic acidosis (decreased pH, negative base excess) in proportion to the severity of illness. An acidosis may also be seen in diabetic ketoacidosis, or surgical patients who lose bicarbonate via the gastrointestinal tract (e.g. diarrhoea, fistulae).

In addition to these values, many modern blood gas analysers will also measure electrolytes and lactate. An increase in the latter implies significant impairment of tissue oxygenation.

Key points:

1 A pulse oximeter does not measure $PaCO_2$ and, therefore, gives no indication of the adequacy of a patient's ventilation.
2 Hypoxaemic patients tend to hyperventilate, with a resultant low $PaCO_2$
3 If a patient is receiving oxygen therapy, the S_pO_2 may be normal, despite inadequate ventilation.
4 A normal PaO_2 (12–14 kPa) whilst breathing 100% oxygen ($FiO_2 = 1.0$) is not normal.

Assessing the circulation (C)

The aim is to identify and treat shock whatever the cause because, if untreated, it will lead to ischaemic damage to the vital organs.

Shock is the inadequate perfusion of the vital organs with oxygenated blood.

In most surgical (and medical) emergencies, the cause of shock is hypovolaemia until proven otherwise. In surgical patients, haemorrhage (overt or hidden) must be rapidly excluded. Respiratory pathology, such as a tension pneumothorax, can also compromise a patient's circulatory state, but will already have been detected and treated if the above system has been followed.

Look:

- At the colour of the hands and digits; are they cyanosed, pale, or mottled, indicating poor peripheral perfusion?
- At the state of the peripheral veins; are they underfilled or collapsed, signifying hypovolaemia, and central veins; are they collapsed or engorged?
- For other signs of a poor cardiac output, for example reduced level of consciousness, oliguria (urine volume <0.5 mL/kg/h).

- For obvious signs of blood or ECF loss; bleeding, nasogastric or other drain loss.
- NOTE: empty drains do not exclude active bleeding. Haemorrhage may be concealed (e.g. intrathoracic, intraperitoneal, pelvic, or into the gut).

Feel:

- Assess limb temperature by feeling the patient's hands and feet. Are they warm, or cool suggesting poor perfusion?
- Measure the capillary refill time (CRT). Apply firm pressure to a finger tip or toe for 5 s (at heart level or just above) and release: the capillaries should refill (colour returns to the compressed area) in <2 s. CRT may be affected by the environmental temperature.
- Palpate a peripheral pulse (usually at the radial artery). Assess for:
  - rate;
  - volume;
  - regularity/rhythm.
- If the radial pulse is absent, assess a central pulse; carotid, brachial, or femoral.
- A weak, thready pulse suggests a poor cardiac output. A bounding pulse may indicate sepsis.

Listen:

- Auscultate the heart. Are there added sounds, for example a third heart sound indicative of heart failure, a murmur of valvular disease, or a pericardial rub suggesting pericarditis?

If not already done, measure the patient's blood pressure, both systolic and diastolic values. Even in shock, the blood pressure may be relatively normal, especially in the young, as compensatory mechanisms increase peripheral resistance in response to reduced cardiac output. There are many causes of hypotension (Table 5.5). Generally, a low DBP suggests arterial vasodilatation (as in anaphylaxis or sepsis); a narrowed pulse pressure (difference between systolic and diastolic pressures; normally about 35–45 mmHg) suggests arterial vasoconstriction (cardiogenic shock or hypovolaemia).

Heart rate and blood pressure must be placed in context; an elderly patient with poor myocardial reserve may be in extemis with a heart rate of 60/min and blood pressure of 95/60 mmHg, but the same values will be well tolerated or even normal for a fit young adult.

Table 5.5 Causes of systemic hypotension.

Causes
Hypovolaemia
• Dehydration/inadequate fluid intake
• Haemorrhage
• Severe vomiting/diarrhoea
• Burns
• Abnormal fluid losses into the gut
• High output fistula of the small bowel
Cardiogenic causes
• Acute myocardial ischaemia/infarction
• Arrhythmias
• Severe valvular heart disease
• Cardiomyopathy
• Acute myocarditis
• Cardiac tamponade
• Constrictive pericarditis
Sepsis
• Any cause of systemic sepsis
Neurogenic
• High spinal cord injury
Anaphylaxis
Others
• Drug overdose

Although ultimately treatment of shock will be determined by the cause, if there are signs and symptoms of shock, the initial response is directed towards:

- Restoration of tissue perfusion with fluid replacement.
- Haemorrhage control.

Nearly all patients who are tachycardic and hypotensive will respond to a fluid challenge. In all cases, obtain venous access (14 or 16 gauge IV cannula). Before connecting the IV fluid, take blood for routine investigations: full blood count, C-reactive protein (CRP), urea, electrolytes, coagulation studies, microbiological investigations, and blood grouping and cross-matching.

Give a rapid fluid challenge (over 5–10 min):

- 500 mL of warmed crystalloid solution, if the patient's SBP is >100 mmHg
- 1000 mL of warmed crystalloid solution, if the patient's SBP is <100 mmHg

• 250 mL of warmed crystalloid solution, if the patient has pre-existing cardiac failure.

Reassess the pulse rate and blood pressure regularly (every 5 min), watching for signs of improvement; decreased pulse rate, increased blood pressure, improved level of consciousness. If not already done, consider inserting a urinary catheter. A urine output of 50–100 mL/h suggests adequate vital organ perfusion.

In patients with known cardiac failure, early consideration should be given to invasive monitoring, for example CVP. Early use of direct arterial pressure measurement is also valuable (see Table 6.3).

If the patient shows no signs of improvement, the fluid challenge can be repeated. Consider the possibility of:

• massive or continuing haemorrhage;
• septic shock;
• cardiac tamponade.

Early expert help is essential in the management of these conditions.

If symptoms and signs of cardiac failure are present or develop (dyspnoea, increased heart rate, raised JVP, a third heart sound, and pulmonary crepitations on auscultation) the rate at which fluid is being given should be reduced or stopped altogether. These patients will often need alternative means of improving tissue perfusion:

• nitrates or diuretics to reduce the high preload to the left ventricle;
• vasodilators to reduce afterload;
• inotropes to increase myocardial contractility.

Such patients will need to be managed in a critical care setting.

Key points:

1 Resting heart rate is normally lower than systolic blood pressure.
2 In some patients, e.g., those with gastro-intestinal or intra-abdominal haemorrhage, immediate surgery may be required as the only effective form of resuscitation.
3 Patients with cardiac failure do just as badly if the heart is underfilled as if it is overfilled and so may benefit from intravenous fluids.

Assessing neurological state—disability (D)

The aim is to assess the patient's conscious level and, if impaired, identify and if possible treat the cause. Common causes of unconsciousness are shown in Table 5.6. Hypoxaemia, hypercapnia, or cerebral hypoperfusion should have been detected and treated at an earlier stage of the ABCDE assessment.

Examine the pupils for size and reactivity to light:

• Pinpoint pupils, reactive: opioids, pontine haemorrhage.
• Mid-sized, fixed: lesion in the midbrain.
• Dilated, fixed: severe ischaemia or hypoxia, hypoglycaemia, brainstem lesion, postseizure, sympathomimetcs (e.g. overdose of tricyclic antidepressant drugs), recent IV administration of adrenaline.
• Unilateral dilatation, fixed: expanding intracranial haematoma causing uncal herniation, lesion of third (oculomotor) cranial nerve.

Check the patient's drug chart for reversible drug-induced causes of depressed consciousness. Give the appropriate antagonist where available, for example naloxone for opioids.

Assess the patient's conscious level using the Glasgow Coma Scale (GCS; see Table 5.7). Record the best response. Measure the blood glucose using

Table 5.6 Common causes of a decreased conscious level.

Hypoxaemia
Hypotension
Hypercapnia
Hypoglycaemia
Hyponatraemia
Drugs (e.g. sedatives, opiates, overdoses)
Seizures
Head injury
Intracranial haemorrhage
Cerebral infarction
Intracranial infection
Cerebral neoplasm
Hypothermia
Hyperthermia
Hypothyroidism
Hepatic encephalopathy

Table 5.7 The Glasgow Coma Scale.

Assessment and response	Score
Eye opening	
Spontaneous	4
To speech	3
To pain	2
None	1
Verbal response	
Orientated	5
Confused	4
Inappropriate words	3
Incomprehensible sounds	2
None	1
Best motor response	
Obeys commands	6
Localizes to pain	5
Withdraws from pain	4
Abnormal flexion to pain	3
Extension to pain	2
None	1

Highest achievable score is 15; the lowest score is 3. Coma is defined as a score of 8 or less; patients have no eye-opening (1), no verbalization (2), and do not obey commands (5).

a rapid bedside method to exclude hypoglycaemia. If below 3 mmol/L, administer 25–50 mL of 50% glucose solution IV.

Key points:

1 Patients with who are in coma (GCS<9) are at risk of airway obstruction when supine and airway reflexes may be insufficient to prevent aspiration of secretions, vomit or blood. Nurse in the recovery position and summon expert help to secure their airway.
2 If there is a risk of co-existing cervical spine pathology e.g. a fracture, nurse the patient supine position maintaining a patent airway. This mandates the constant presence of a nurse or doctor.

Exposure/examination (E)

The aim is to allow a full, head-to-toe, back and front examination of the patient. To allow this, full exposure of the body is necessary, carried out in a way that respects the dignity of the patient and prevents heat loss. Initially, the examination should be focused on the area of the body most likely to be causing the patient's condition; for example, for a patient presenting with shock following a laparotomy, this would be the abdomen.

What to do next?

The aim of the interventions so far has been to keep the patient alive and produce some clinical improvement, to enable a diagnosis to be made and definitive treatment initiated. Even if the patient's vital signs are still outside the normal range, they should be moving in a direction of improvement. If not, it is essential to summon senior help and, while waiting for them to arrive, reassess the patient using the ABCDE approach to identify the cause.

Once things are improving, gather more information about the patient:

- Take a full history from the patient, staff, or the notes. Comorbid conditions (e.g. ischaemic heart disease, COPD) can have a significant impact upon a patient's response to critical illness, and must not be overlooked.
- If not already done, perform a full examination of the patient, using a traditional clinical examination format.
- Review the patient's notes and charts. Assimilate the data on charts by systematic analysis. Study both absolute values of vital signs and their trends.
- Check that important routine medications are prescribed and being administered. Look for potential interactions.
- Review the results of all laboratory and radiological investigations.

Consider if you have a credible diagnosis that accounts for the patient's condition and recent deterioration:

- If yes, consider the definitive treatment of the patient's underlying condition.
- If no, re-assess the patient in case you have missed something important. Involve more senior colleagues.

Consider which level of care is required by the patient (e.g. ward, HDU, ICU). This may be dictated by your hospital's policies.

Make complete entries in the patient's notes of your finding, assessment, and treatment. Record the patient's response to therapy. Make sure that your entry in the notes is legible, signed, dated, and timed.

Communicating information about patient deterioration

Although the systems outlined above will allow the recognition, initial assessment, and treatment of the acutely ill patient, on the majority of occasions, more senior help will be required to manage the problem safely and effectively. The key to achieving this is good communication at all levels:

Know why you are calling before picking up the phone.

- Do you want a more senior colleague to assess the patient?
- Are you calling for advice?
- Do you think the patient needs an operation?
- Before making the call, gather all the useful information together.
- Be assertive when communicating, avoid aggression, and be honest. 'I am unsure of what to do next' or 'I am worried that I am missing something' are likely to assist in obtaining help.

Get the message across in the first two sentences:

- 'This is . . . I am sorry to disturb you, but Mr Smith is deteriorating and I think that he may need an urgent operation'.

Key point:

Use a system for communicating patient deterioration, for example RSVP.
R = Reason for calling
S = Story
V= Vital signs (plus any early warning score)
P = Plan

Critical care outreach services

Amongst its recommendations, the 2000 document, 'Comprehensive Critical Care', stressed that patient care on general wards could be improved if critical care areas (i.e. ICUs and HDUs) shared their skills with general ward staff. This concept recognizes that the vast majority of patients are on the general wards of hospitals when they start to deteriorate and not in a critical care unit, and that critical care is a process rather than a place. Many hospitals now have 'outreach teams', usually consisting of one or more nurses along with a doctor trained in critical care.

Outreach services have three essential objectives:

- To avert admissions by identifying patients who are deteriorating and intervene either to help prevent admission or to ensure that admission to a critical care bed happens in a timely manner to ensure the best outcome.
- To enable discharges from critical care by supporting the continuing recovery of discharged patients on wards and after discharge from hospital.
- To share critical care skills with staff on wards, in the community, enhance training opportunities and skills, and to gather feedback to improve critical care services for patients and relatives.

If your hospital has an outreach service, you will find it useful in supporting you in the care of your patients with critical illness.

Cardiac arrest

Unfortunately, significant numbers of patients in hospital will have a cardiac arrest either as a result of primary cardiac disease or as the end point of unrecognized physiological deterioration. All healthcare professionals need to be competent with dealing with a patient who has a cardiac arrest, either as a first responder or as a member of the cardiac arrest team.

In-hospital cardiac arrest management (Fig. 5.2)

On discovering a collapsed patient in a clinical area:

- Shout for help.
- Ensure personal safety:
  - Check immediate surroundings are safe.
  - Put on gloves as soon as available.

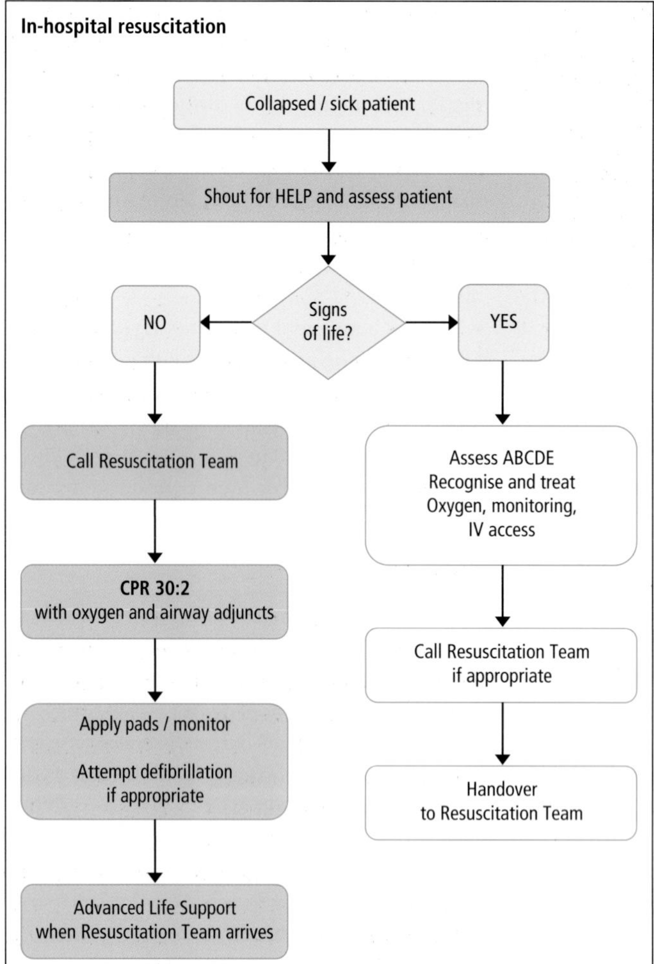

Figure 5.2 The algorithm for in-hospital cardiac arrest. Courtesy of the Resuscitation Council (UK).

  - Use a pocket mask with a filter to reduce risk of transmission of infection.
  - Correct disposal of 'sharps'.
  - Avoid mouth-to-mouth if poisons or chemicals are involved.
- Assess the patient's responsiveness, 'Are you alright?'
- Confirm cardiac arrest:
  - Look, listen, feel for breathing for up to 10 s; if trained to do so, check for a carotid pulse.
- If alone, call the cardiac arrest team, and on return start cardiopulmonary resuscitation (CPR).
- If two persons are present:
  - No. 1 starts CPR, 30 compressions followed by two ventilations.
  - No. 2 calls the cardiac arrest team and collects resuscitation equipment and a defibrillator.
- When the equipment arrives:
  - Attach monitor/defibrillator or automated external defibrillator (AED) as soon as possible.
  - Defibrillate if trained to do so; do not delay for ventilations or chest compressions.
- Hand over to the cardiac arrest team leader when the team arrives.
- If not trained to use an AED, continue CPR until the cardiac arrest team arrives

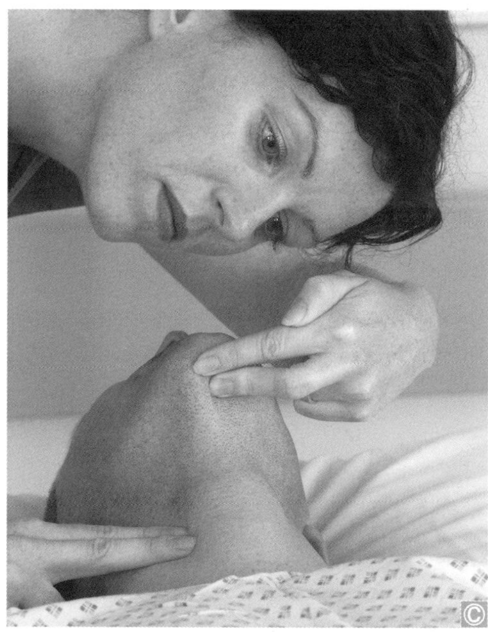

Figure 5.3 Look, listen, and feel for evidence of breathing while checking the carotid pulse.

Airway and ventilation

Most patients who suffer a cardiac arrest will have an obstructed airway. The basic airway opening manoeuvres of a head tilt and chin lift should be used to provide a clear airway, while simultaneously a check for a carotid pulse can be made (Fig. 5.3). Insertion of an LMA (Fig. 3.8) will provide a more secure airway. Use a jaw thrust with manual in-line stabilization of the head and neck (Fig 5.4) if there is any possibility of injury to the cervical spine. The patient can then be ventilated using a self-inflating bag, either via a facemask (Fig. 5.1) or via the LMA. Tracheal intubation should only be attempted by those trained and competent to do so. Whichever technique is used, supplementary oxygen should be given as soon as available. An inspiratory time of 1 s should be used and sufficient volume given to see the chest rise. Inadequate ventilation is usually due to: an obstructed airway because of failure to maintain head tilt or jaw thrust, leaks around the facemask or LMA, or an unrecognized foreign body in the airway.

Chest compressions

At best this only generates a cardiac output about 25% of normal and, in order to achieve this, the correct technique is essential. The correct position for the hands is the middle of the lower half of the sternum (Fig. 5.5). The heel of one hand is placed in position and the second hand placed on the back of the first, with the fingers interlocked. The sternum is compressed to a depth of 4–5 cm, followed by complete release of pressure. This is repeated at a rate of 100/min, with compression and relaxation taking the same period of time. To

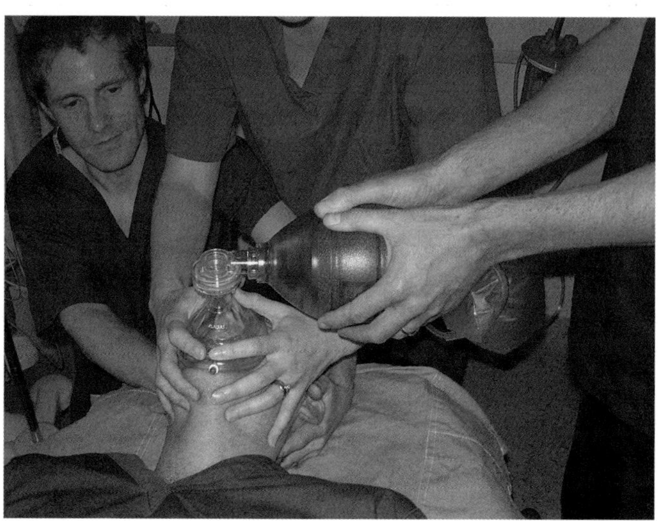

Figure 5.4 Ventilation with a self-inflating bag-valve-mask using the two-person technique, with application of manual in-line stabilization in a patient with potential cervical spine injury.

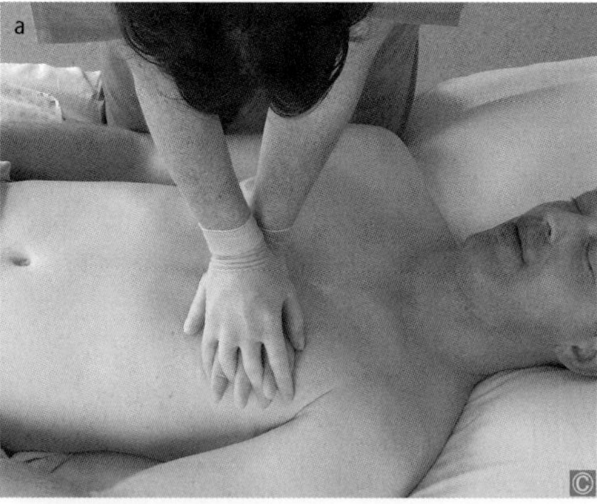

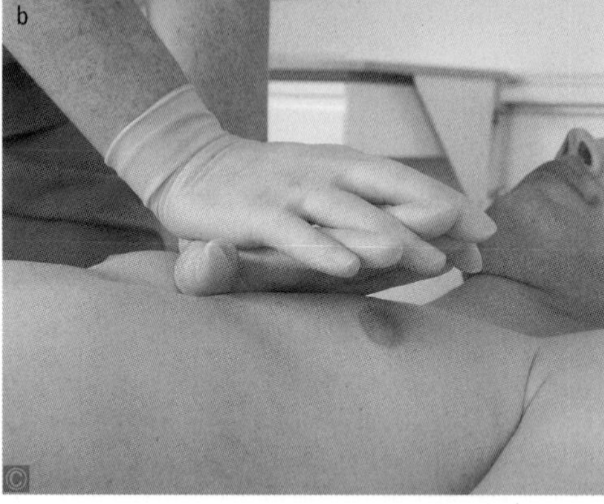

Figure 5.5 Chest compressions during CPR.

optimize compressions and reduce rescuer fatigue, chest compressions are best performed with the rescuer leaning well forward over the patient, arms straight, and hands, arms, and shoulders in a straight line. This allows use of the performer's upper body weight to achieve compressions rather than the arm muscles that will tire rapidly and reduce efficacy.

Common errors

Wrong hand position:
- too high: the heart is not compressed;
- too low: the stomach is compressed and risk of aspiration increased;
- too laterally: injures underlying organs, for example liver, spleen, bowel.

Overenthusiastic effort:
- causes cardiac damage;
- fractures ribs which may damage underlying organs, particularly lungs and liver.

Inadequate effort:
- the rescuer is not high enough above the patient to use his/her body weight;
- fatigue during prolonged resuscitation or because of poor technique.

Failure to release between compressions:
- prevents venous return and filling of the heart.

Automated external defibrillators (AEDs)

These are defibrillators that have the capacity to analyse the cardiac rhythm and give either visual or voice prompts or both that a shock is required. When this is the case, the machine will usually charge automatically, and the shock is delivered when the operator presses the appropriate button. Some devices are fully automated and deliver the shock once charged. It is essential that while the machine is analysing the waveform, nobody touches the patient as this will delay the process. Training in the use of an AED is easier than for a manual device, allows a greater number of individuals in hospital to defibrillate, reduces the time to first defibrillation, and increases the number of people who survive to discharge from hospital after cardiac arrest.

Advanced life support

Advance life support (ALS) management is summarized in Fig. 5.6. The interested reader should refer to the Resuscitation Council (UK) website for further details.

Shockable rhythms

The onset of ventricular fibrillation (VF) may be preceded by a period of pulseless ventricular tachycardia (VT). The most effective treatment of *both conditions* is identical—electrical defibrillation (a direct current, DC, shock). The time to delivery of the first shock is critical in determining the outcome and, therefore, once the diagnosis has been made, defibrillation is the first manoeuvre to

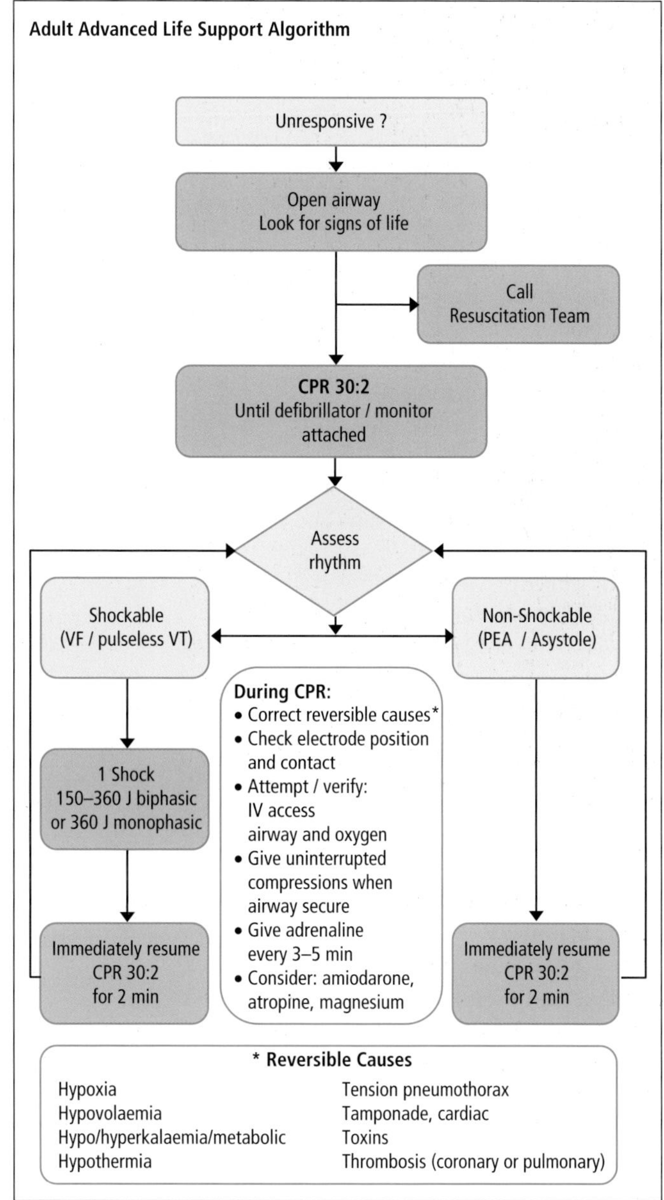

Figure 5.6 Adult Advance Life Support algorithm. Courtesy of the Resuscitation Council (UK).

be carried out in ALS. The only exception to this is when it is preceded by a precordial thump. This manoeuvre should only be used if the cardiac arrest was witnessed and/or monitored. A sharp blow is delivered to the patient's sternum with a closed fist. This delivers a small amount of mechanical energy to the myocardium and, if done early enough after the onset of VF, may cause the rhythm to revert to one capable of restoring the circulation.

The sequence of treating VF/VT

- Confirm rhythm is VF/VT
- Defibrillate using a single shock of 150–200 J if biphasic, 360 J if monophasic.

- Immediately restart CPR without checking for a pulse or reassessing the rhythm
- Continue CPR for 2 min.
- After 2 min, pause briefly to check the monitor.
- If VF/VT persists:
  - Give second shock, 150–360 J biphasic, 360 J monophasic.
  - Immediately restart CPR for 2 min.
  - After 2 min, pause briefly to check the monitor.
- If VF/VT persists:
  - Give 1 mg of adrenaline IV.
  - Follow immediately by third shock, 150–360 J biphasic, 360 J monophasic.
  - Immediately restart CPR for 2 min.
  - After 2 min, pause briefly to check the monitor.
- If VF/VT persists:
  - Give 300 mg of amiodarone IV.
  - Follow immediately by fourth shock, 150–360 J biphasic, 360 J monophasic.
  - Immediately restart CPR for 2 min.
  - Give 1 mg of adrenaline IV immediately before alternative shocks, approximately every 3–5 min.
  - Give further shocks after each 2 min period of CPR while VF/VT persists.

Points to note

- Do not take more than 10 s from stopping CPR to delivering the shock. Coronary artery blood flow falls rapidly as CPR ceases and reduces the chance of successful defibrillation.
- Even if the shock is successful in treating VF/VT, it is unlikely that a pulse will be palpable immediately. Continuing CPR does not increase the risk of VF recurring. If a perfusing rhythm has not been restored, checking for a pulse simply wastes time.
- Do not delay defibrillation; if the adrenaline is not ready, give it after the shock.
- Do not interrupt chest compressions to check for a pulse unless the patient shows signs of life.
- If the rhythm changes to asystole or PEA, change to the non-shockable side of the algorithm.

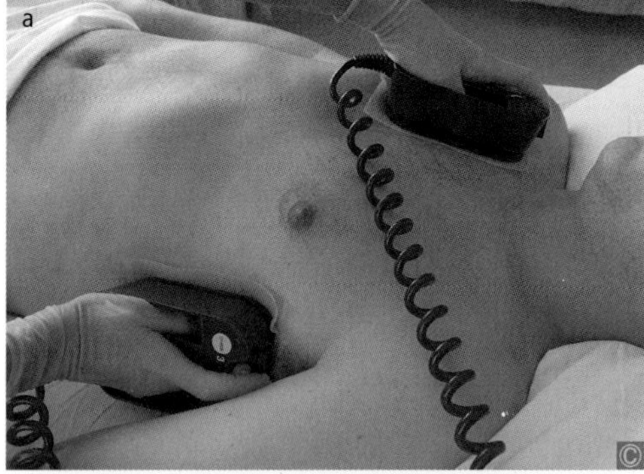

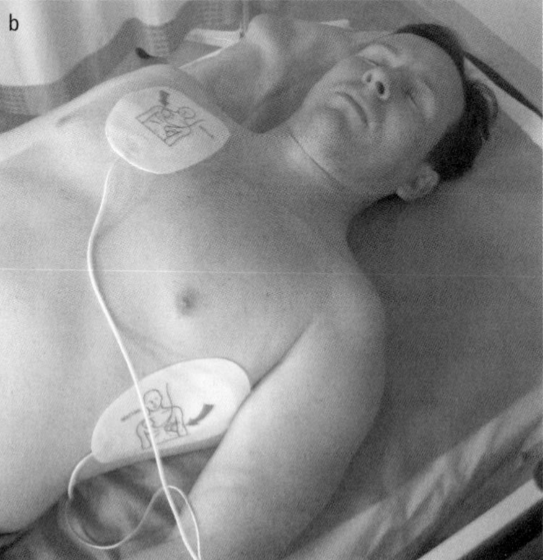

Figure 5.7 (a) Paddle and (b) pad position for external cardiac defibrillation.

Defibrillation

The self-adhesive electrodes or gel-pads and paddles are placed anterolateral: one to the right of the sternum, just below the clavicle; and the other over the apex, below and to the left of the nipple. Although they may be marked positive and negative, each can be placed in either position (Fig. 5.7a, b). An alternative is to place them anteroposterior to the heart.

Safe defibrillation

The discharge of a defibrillator delivers enough current to cause as well as to treat VF; therefore safety is paramount when performing defibrillation:

- Turn on the power switch (ensure the synchronization switch is set to 'OFF').
- Put self-adhesive pads or gel-pads and paddles on patient's chest and press firmly into place.
- Select correct energy level.
- Check oxygen has been removed.
- Warn team members that you are charging the defibrillator.
- Charge the defibrillator.
- Shout 'stand back' and make a visual check of the area.
- Perform a final check of patient's ECG rhythm.
- Deliver shock.
- Restart CPR without checking for a pulse.
- Replace paddles in the defibrillator.

If using gel-pads and paddles, remember:

- It is essential that the defibrillator is charged only when the paddles are on the patient's chest and must not be moved between defibrillator and patient whilst charged.
- Ensure that the paddles are not touching when on the chest, or connected by misplaced gel-pads, as this will cause arcing on discharge, insufficient current delivery, and the patient to be burned.
- Gel-pads can result in the spurious diagnosis of asystole after several shocks have been given due to poor conductivity.

Self-adhesive electrodes avoid the above problems, allow hands-free defibrillation, keep the operator at a safe distance from the patient rather than leaning over them, and for these reasons are preferable to paddles.

Whichever device is used, the operator must ensure that nobody else is in contact with the patient or trolley, directly or indirectly (via spilt electrolyte solution), when the defibrillator is discharged. Any nitrate patches should be removed from the patient's chest along with any high-flow oxygen to eliminate the risk of fire. Finally, a clear verbal warning, usually a shout of 'stand back', and a visual check of the area are mandatory before discharging the defibrillator. If the defibrillator has been charged in error while the paddles or electrodes are on the patient, most devices will allow the charge to be 'dumped' safely by changing the energy level setting.

Waveform characteristics

With older defibrillators, the current passes from one paddle to the other and the waveform is described as being monophasic. These devices are no longer manufactured, but many are still in use. All modern defibrillators now deliver a biphasic waveform in which the current flow is reversed half way through its delivery. This waveform is more effective at treating VF and, as lower energies are used, smaller batteries and capacitors can be used. When combined with solid-state circuitry rather than an inductor to control the waveform, modern biphasic defibrillators are smaller, lighter, and more portable.

Synchronized defibrillation

Defibrillation can be attempted at any point on the VF waveform (an unsynchronized shock). However, when the rhythm is pulseless VT, the shock should be delivered on the 'r' wave, i.e. synchronized. This may also be referred to as cardioversion. If the shock is delivered on the 't' wave, when the heart is refractory, then VF may be precipitated. Some defibrillators automatically default to synchronized mode when switched on, and unless cancelled this may delay delivery of a shock if the patient is in VF.

Non-shockable rhythms—asystole and pulseless electrical activity (PEA)

Asystole

This represents electrical standstill of the heart with no contractile activity, and is seen on the ECG as a gently undulating baseline. It is essential to rule out the possibility of VF having been misdiagnosed before the diagnosis of asystole is made, consequently:

- check equipment function;
- ensure that the ECG leads are connected;
- check the gain setting;
- check the lead setting, lead I or II.

If there is any doubt about the diagnosis, treatment should begin as for VF. The risks of not treating VF are greater than that of an unnecessary shock. A precordial thump can be used under the same criteria as for VF. Occasionally, if monitoring the patient's rhythm via the paddles, 'spurious' asystole may be seen after the delivery of a shock (more likely when successive sequences of shocks have been delivered via the same pads). It is essential that the rhythm is confirmed rapidly using ECG electrodes. In general, the outcome from asystole is poor unless there are 'p' waves present that may respond to cardiac pacing.

PEA

This is the term used to describe the situation when there are recognizable complexes on the ECG compatible with a cardiac output but the patient is pulseless. It is usually a result of conditions that mechanically restrict cardiac filling or outflow, or biochemically disrupt cardiac contractility. Common causes are listed in the ALS algorithm (Fig 5.6). The patient's best chance of survival is rapid identification and treatment of the underlying cause.

Drugs used during ALS

Adrenaline

This is a naturally occurring catecholamine, administered during CPR for its profound alpha-agonist (vasoconstrictor) properties. This leads to an increase in the peripheral vascular resistance that tends to divert blood flow to the vital organs (heart, brain). It is the first drug used in cardiac arrest of any aetiology. The adult dose is 1 mg IV, i.e. 1 mL of 1 : 1000 or 10 mL of 1 : 10 000, administered during ALS every 3–5 min. If IV access cannot be obtained, larger doses (2–3 mg) can be administered via a tracheal tube diluted to 10 mL with sterile water.

Amiodarone

The main indication for this drug in cardiac arrest is during shock-refractory VF or pulseless VT, when it should be given immediately before the delivery of the fourth shock. The adult dose in cardiac arrest is 300 mg, diluted to 20 mL and given preferably via a central line, or alternatively a peripheral line.

Atropine

An anticholinergic drug that acts at muscarinic receptors. It blocks the vagus nerve at both the sinoatrial (SA) and atrioventricular (AV) nodes, causing an increase in heart rate. In cardiac arrest due to asystole or PEA where the heart rate is less than 60 beats/min, the adult dose is 3 mg IV. A dose of 6 mg can be given via a tracheal tube.

Open chest cardiac compression

The output generated by direct compression of the heart is two to three times greater than closed chest compression, and coronary and cerebral perfusion pressures are significantly higher. The procedure is performed via a left thoracotomy through the fourth or fifth intercostal space. It is of most use following penetrating trauma, but unlikely to benefit those in which cardiac arrest follows blunt trauma. It can also be considered in those patients in whom closed chest compression is less effective, namely severe emphysema, a rigid chest wall, severe valvular heart disease, or recent sternotomy. There is no evidence to support its use as a routine procedure.

Paediatric basic life support

The general principles are the same as for adult basic life support, but specific techniques are required to take into account the altered anatomy and physiology of children. Furthermore, if the optimum support is to be given, the techniques must be adjusted according to the size of the child. 'Infant' is used to mean those less than 1 year old, and children to indicate those between 1 year and puberty.

The evaluation of the victim is as for adults, accepting that infants and very small children who cannot yet talk, and older children who are very scared, are unlikely to reply meaningfully, but they may make some sound or open their eyes to the rescuer's voice.

The algorithm for paediatric basic life support for healthcare professionals with a duty to respond is shown in Fig 5.8.

- Ensure personal and child's safety:
  - Check immediate surroundings are safe.
  - Put on gloves as soon as available.
  - Use a pocket mask with a filter to reduce risk of transmission of infection.

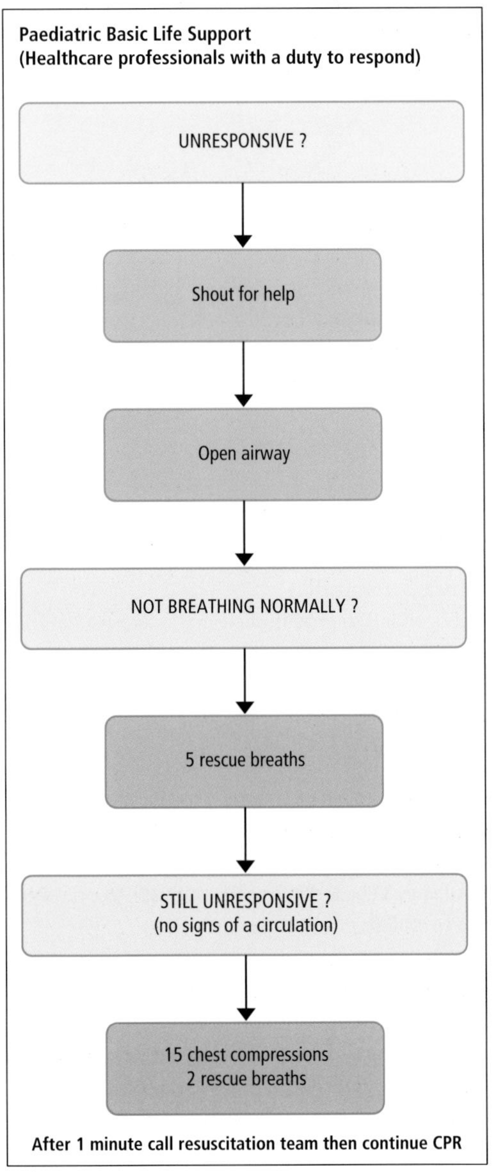

Figure 5.8 The algorithm for paediatric basic life support (BLS) algorithm. Courtesy of the Resuscitation Council (UK).

  - Avoid mouth-to-mouth if poisons or chemicals are involved.
- Assess the child's responsiveness, stimulate and ask loudly 'Are you alright?'
- Confirm cardiac arrest:
  - Open the airway, look, listen, feel for breathing for up to 10 s.
- If not breathing normally (apnoeic or agonal gasps):
  - Remove obvious obstructions.
  - Give 5 rescue breaths.
- Check for signs of a circulation (no more than 10 s):
  - Infant; brachial pulse medial aspect of upper arm.
  - Child; carotid pulse.
- If no signs of a circulation (or bradycardia (<60 beats/min) and poor perfusion):
  - Give 15 chest compressions, at a rate of 100/min.
  - Continue compressions and breaths at a ratio of 15 : 2.
- If alone, after 1 min, call the cardiac arrest team, and on return continue CPR.
- Lone rescuers may use a ratio of 30:2 if difficult moving from compressions to ventilations.
- If two persons are present:
  - No. 1 starts compressions followed by ventilations.
  - No. 2 calls the cardiac arrest team and collects resuscitation equipment and a defibrillator.
- In a witnessed arrest, even a single rescuer must get help before starting resuscitation.
- When the victim is an infant or small child, it may be possible to carry them to the point where help is summoned to minimize interruptions in CPR.
- When the equipment arrives:
  - Attach monitor/defibrillator or AED as soon as possible.
  - Defibrillate if trained to do so; do not delay for ventilations or chest compressions.
- Hand over to the cardiac arrest team leader when the team arrives.
- If not trained to use an AED, continue CPR until the cardiac arrest team arrives.

Airway control

If the child is not breathing, it may be because the airway has been blocked by the tongue falling back to obstruct the pharynx. Correction of this problem may result in recovery without further intervention.

• *Head tilt plus chin lift* A hand is placed on the forehead, and the head is gently tilted back as for an adult. In an infant, the tilt should be just sufficient to place the head in a neutral position. The fingers of the other hand should then be placed under the chin, lifting it upwards. Care should be taken not to injure the soft tissue by gripping too hard. It may be necessary to use the thumb of the same hand to part the lips slightly.

• *Jaw thrust* This is most appropriate for children and achieved by placing two or three fingers under the angle of the mandible bilaterally, and lifting the jaw upwards. It may be easier if the rescuer's elbows are resting on the same surface as the child is lying on. A small degree of head tilt may also be applied.

The finger sweep technique often recommended for adults should not be used in children. The child's soft palate is easily damaged, causing bleeding, and foreign bodies may become impacted in the child's cone-shaped airway and be even more difficult to remove.

Breathing

The airway is kept open using the techniques described above. If the mouth of the child alone is used, then the nose should be pinched closed using the thumb and index fingers of the hand that is maintaining the head tilt. In infants and small children, mouth-to-mouth and nose ventilation should be used. Each breath should last 1–1.5 s, providing sufficient volume to make the child's chest rise. Since children vary in size, only general guidance can be given regarding the volume and pressure of inflation:

• the chest should be seen to rise and fall;

• inflation pressures may be relatively high as the airways are smaller;

• slow breaths at the lowest pressure reduce gastric distension;

If the chest does not rise then the airway is not clear:

• readjust the head tilt/chin lift position;

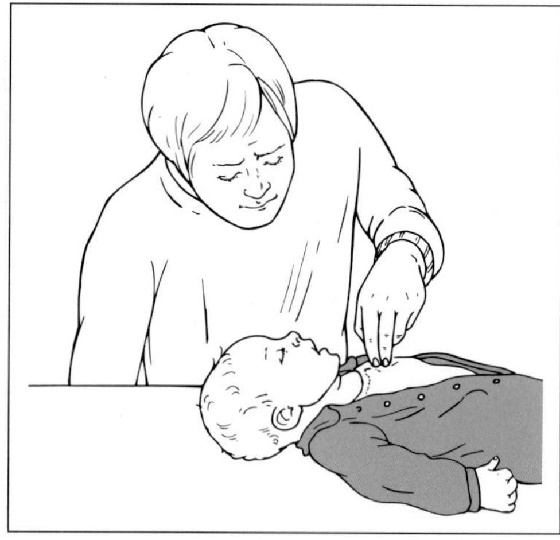

Figure 5.9 Infant chest compressions.

• try a jaw thrust;

• if both fail to provide a clear airway, suspect that a foreign body is causing obstruction.

Circulation

In children of all ages, compress the lower third of the sternum. Locate the xiphisternum and compress one finger's breadth above this. The force used should be sufficient to compress to one-third the overall depth of the child's chest.

Infants

The lone rescuer should compress the sternum with the tips of two adjacent fingers (Fig. 5.9). If there are two or more rescuers, use the hand-encircling technique. The infant is held with both the rescuer's hands encircling the chest. The thumbs are placed over the correct part of the sternum (see above) and compression carried out.

Children over 1 year

Place the heel of one hand over the lower third of the sternum. Ensure fingers are raised so that the chest is not compressed (Fig. 5.10). For small rescuers or in large children, a two-handed technique with fingers interlocked may be necessary to achieve the correct compression.

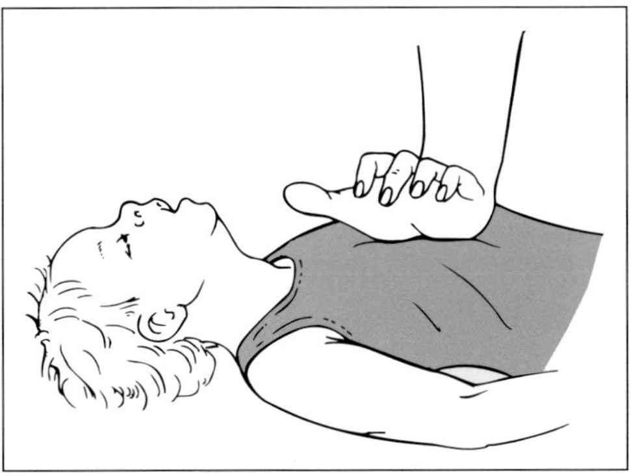

Figure 5.10 Child chest compressions—one hand.

Automated external defibrillators

- A standard AED can be used in children over 8 years.
- There are specific pads or programs for the energy output from a standard AED to allow it to be used for children between 1 and 8 years.
- If such equipment or a manually adjustable defibrillator is not available, an unmodified adult AED can be used for children over 1 year.

Education in acute care

Recently, there has been increasing concern about the adequacy of training, and the resulting level of knowledge and skills possessed by healthcare professionals in recognizing and treating an acutely ill patient. Data suggest that many staff do not possess the necessary competencies to detect acute illness and safely manage acutely ill patients. Additionally, many also lack confidence in dealing with acute clinical conditions.

In an attempt to counter these problems, several multiprofessional courses that teach a pre-emptive approach to critical illness, for example the Acute Life-threatening Events Recognition and Treatment course (ALERT™), have been developed. At the same time, the competencies required by medical undergraduates have been defined by the Acute Care Undergraduate Teaching (ACUTE) project team, and similar recommendations are currently being developed by the Department of Health for other staff.

The Resuscitation Council (UK) ALS course provides a standardized approach to CPR in adults. The course is aimed at all healthcare professionals who are expected to perform ALS both in and out of hospital. As it is multidisciplinary, all those participating are given the opportunity to function both as team members and as team leaders. For many specialties, completion of the ALS course is a mandatory part of training. The Advanced Paediatric Life Support (APLS) course covers the management of the critically ill or injured child.

Further reading

Andrews T, Waterman H. Packaging: a grounded theory of how to report physiological deterioration effectively. *Journal of Advanced Nursing* 2005; **52**: 473–81.

DeVita MA, Bellomo R, Hillman K, *et al*. Findings of the first consensus conference on medical emergency teams. *Critical Care Medicine* 2006; **34**: 2463–78.

Driscoll P, Brown T, Gwinnutt C, Wardle T. *A simple guide to blood gas analysis*. London: BMJ Publishing Group, 1997.

Esmonde L, McDonnell A, Ball C *et al*. Investigating the effectiveness of critical care outreach services: a systematic review. *Intensive Care Medicine* 2006; **32**: 1713–21.

Gao H, McDonnell A, Harrison DA *et al*. Systematic review and evaluation of physiological track and trigger warning systems for identifying at-risk patients on the ward. *Intensive Care Medicine* 2007; **33**: 667–79.

Hodgetts TJ, Kenward G, Vlackonikolis I *et al*. Incidence, location and reasons for avoidable in-hospital cardiac arrest in a district general hospital. *Resuscitation* 2002; **54**: 115–23.

Kause J, Smith G, Prytherch D, Parr M, Flabouris A, Hillman K. A comparison of antecedents to cardiac arrests, deaths and emergency intensive care admissions in Australia and New Zealand, and the United Kingdom—the ACADEMIA study. *Resuscitation* 2004; **62**: 275–82.

McDonnell A, Esmonde L, Morgan R *et al.* The provision of critical care outreach services in England: findings from a national survey. *Journal of Critical Care* 2007; **22**: 212–18.

McGloin H, Adam SK, Singer M. Unexpected deaths and referrals to intensive care of patients on general wards. Are some cases potentially avoidable? *Journal of the Royal College of Physicians of London* 1999; **33**: 255–9.

McQuillan P, Pilkington S, Allan A *et al.* Confidential inquiry into quality of care before admission to intensive care. *British Medical Journal* 1998; **316**: 1853–8.

Perkins GD, Barrett H, Bullock I *et al.* The Acute Care Undergraduate TEaching (ACUTE) initiative: consensus development of core competencies in acute care for undergraduates in the United Kingdom. *Intensive Care Medicine* 2005; **31**: 1627–33.

Smith GB, Osgood VM, Crane S. ALERT—a multiprofessional training course in the care of the acutely ill adult patient. *Resuscitation* 2002; **52**: 281–6.

Smith GB, Poplett N. Knowledge of aspects of acute care in trainee doctors. *Postgraduate Medical Journal* 2002; **78**: 335–8.

Winters BD, Pham JC, Hunt EA, Guallar E, Berenholtz S, Pronovost PJ. Rapid response systems: a systematic review. *Critical Care Medicine* 2007; **35**: 1238–43.

Useful websites

http://www.dh.gov.uk/en/Publicationsandstatistics/Publications/PublicationsPolicyAndGuidance/DH_4006585

[Comprehensive Critical Care. A review of critical care services. Department of Health. 2000.]

http://www.ncepod.org.uk/2005.htm

['An acute problem?'. Published in 2005 by the National Confidential Enquiry into Patient Outcome and Death.]

http://www.nice.org.uk/guidance/index.jsp?action=byID&o=11810

[Recognition of and response to acute illness in adults in hospital. July 2007. The NICE guidelines—you must read this if you are interested in this topic.]

http://www.resus.org.uk/

[The Resuscitation Council UK. This site contains the current UK guidelines for cardiopulmonary resuscitation.]

http://www.erc.edu/

[European Resuscitation Council website.]

http://www.c2005.org/

[This site contains all the scientific data supporting the current guidelines for cardiopulmonary resuscitation.]

http://www.bestbets.org/

[This website contains best evidence topic reviews for emergency medicine. Many of these are relevant to anaesthesia and critically ill patients.]

http://www.sign.ac.uk/guidelines/fulltext/63/index.html

[The British Thoracic Society (BTS) & Scottish Intercollegiate Guidelines Network (SIGN). British Guidelines on the Management of Asthma. February 2003.]

All websites last accessed April 2008.

Self-assessment

5.1 How would you assess a patient for signs of airway obstruction? What would be your immediate management of this problem?

5.2 Define shock. How would you assess a patient for the signs of shock? What would be your immediate management of this problem?

5.3 A 22-year-old male is brought to the Emergency Department by ambulance having been found unconscious on a local park bench. He does not respond when you speak to him, but on applying pressure to his supraorbital ridge, he opens his eyes, says odd words, and tries to push your hand away. On examination of his pupils with a pen torch they are 1.5 mm in diameter. What would be your initial assessment and management of this patient?

5.4 You are called to a medical ward to see a patient who has suddenly deteriorated and is now unresponsive. When you arrive what are your immediate actions?

5.5 What is the sequence of events in the first 6–8 minutes when treating a patient found to be in ventricular fibrillation?

Chapter 6

Management of the critically ill patient

Critically ill patients have a high morbidity and mortality. Prompt recognition and early appropriate management of such patients helps both to minimize further deterioration and to maximize the chances of recovery. However, it is equally important to identify and monitor closely those patients who are at risk of becoming critically ill. In 2000, The Department of Health (UK) published standards for the provision and organization of hospital care for critically ill patients and those at risk of developing critical illness. This proposed a shift in emphasis away from defining the needs of such patients in terms of hospital geography (ICU, HDU, etc.) and towards a classification system that describes escalating levels of care for individual patients, independent of their location within the hospital (Table 6.1). Although this approach does not obviate the requirement for ICUs and HDUs, it does envisage less direct focus on these areas towards a more generalized, hospital-wide approach.

One of the key benefits envisaged by this reorganization of care of critically ill patients is a reduction in referral patterns to ICU and HDU by earlier recognition of warning signs that often presage the development of critical illness and cardiac arrest, thereby prompting earlier initiation of resuscitation and treatment—the so-called 'intensive care without walls' philosophy. The necessary prerequisites for the successful implementation of this integrated approach to the organization of provision of care for critically ill patients are summarized in Table 6.2 and described in more detail below.

'Critical care is a process, not a location'

The intensive care unit—an overview

The ICU is a designated area within a hospital where specialized treatment of critically ill patients takes place (Level 3 care, Fig. 6.1). In order to achieve this, there is a concentration of resources, including:

- a wide range of complex monitoring equipment;
- mechanical ventilators;
- facilities for organ support;
- the use of potent drugs, which are often given by continuous IV infusion;
- a high nurse to patient ratio, typically 1 : 1;
- a medical resident who is continuously available exclusively for the ICU.

The service is consultant-led, i.e. consultants (predominantly anaesthetists in the UK at present) are closely involved with all day-to-day management of critically ill patients, and with supervising, directing, and training nurses and doctors. The out-of-hours commitment of such consultants is onerous as they are normally present on the ICU to supervise directly the initial management of all

Table 6.1 Levels of care for critically ill patients.

Level 0
• Stable patients whose needs can be met through routine ward care
Level 1
• Patients at risk of their condition deteriorating who require careful clinical observation achievable on a general ward
• Patients recently relocated from higher levels of care whose needs can be met with additional advice and support from the critical care team
Level 2 (HDU)
• Patients requiring more detailed monitoring (e.g. invasive arterial blood pressure, CVP)
• Support for a single organ system failure, including non-invasive positive pressure ventilation
• Certain postoperative patients (e.g. after major surgery in high-risk patients)
• Patients stepping down from level 3 care
Level 3 (ICU)
• Patients requiring advanced respiratory support (tracheal intubation and mechanical ventilation)
• Patients with MOFS

Adapted from *Comprehensive Critical Care: a review of adult critical care services*. Department of Health, 2000. Reproduced with permission of the Controller of HMSO.

Table 6.2 Key features of an integrated approach to the provision and organization of care of critically ill patients.

• Earlier recognition of the deteriorating condition of susceptible patients
• Earlier initiation of appropriate treatment/resuscitation
• Earlier referral of patients to the critical care team
• Extension of the resources of the ICU/HDU beyond their geographical limits
These aims may be facilitated by the introduction of:
• Improved training and education of clinical ward staff
• Doctors
• Nurses
• Healthcare assistants
• Use of clinical early warning scoring systems
• Provision of an outreach team

newly referred critically ill patients, admissions to the ICU, and interhospital ICU transfers.

Complementing, or in lieu of, the ICU, there is usually an HDU where the level of care is intermediate (Level 2) between that found on the ICU and the general ward. Patients on the HDU are not normally ventilated via a tracheal tube although they may be non-invasively ventilated (see later). Patients suffering from acute MI are generally admitted to specialized CCUs, while neurosurgical and head-injured patients may be admitted to a specialized area of the neurosurgical ward for short periods of mechanical ventilation. Other specialized HDUs include liver, renal, and burns units.

The challenge for those involved in the care of critically ill patients is to focus precious resources on those patients likely to survive, by providing artificial support of one or more failing physiological systems until natural recuperation and/or therapeutically assisted recovery can take place. Patients may be admitted to the ICU electively following major surgery, or as medical or surgical emergencies. In an attempt to differentiate potential survivors from non-survivors, a number of scoring systems have been developed which take into account various aspects of the patient's acute physiological upset, age, and any chronic health problems (e.g. APACHE II—Acute Physiology and Chronic Health Evaluation). However, none of these scoring systems is accurate enough to be used as the sole basis for deciding whether or not to treat an *individual* patient. Ultimately, there is no substitute for the clinical judgement of an experienced senior intensivist, usually in discussion with the patient's referring consultant.

Monitoring

Physiological monitoring is an essential aid in the diagnosis and management of critically ill patients, in evaluating their response to treatment and

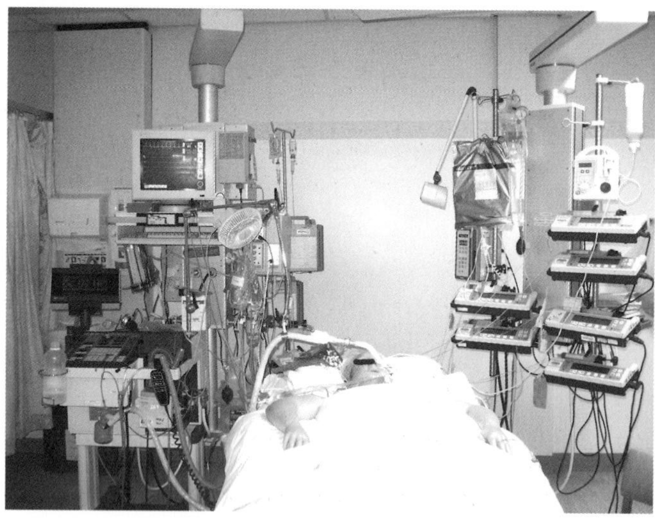

Figure 6.1 Typical view of an ICU patient to show the large amount of equipment required. Ventilator and monitors are on the patient's right; syringe pumps delivering drugs are on the left.

alerting staff to the onset of a sudden deterioration in the patient's condition. There is a spectrum of monitoring. At its most basic level it comprises clinical observation and examination (which, although 'low technology', remains of paramount importance), extending to complex, invasive methods for the measurement of haemodynamics, oxygen transport, and other variables (Fig. 6.2).

Electrocardiogram (ECG)

All patients should have a continuously displayed ECG for the detection of acute dysrhythmias and, to a lesser extent (except on the CCU), acute ischaemia. In critically ill patients on the general ICU, supraventricular tachycardias predominate, especially sinus tachycardia and atrial fibrillation.

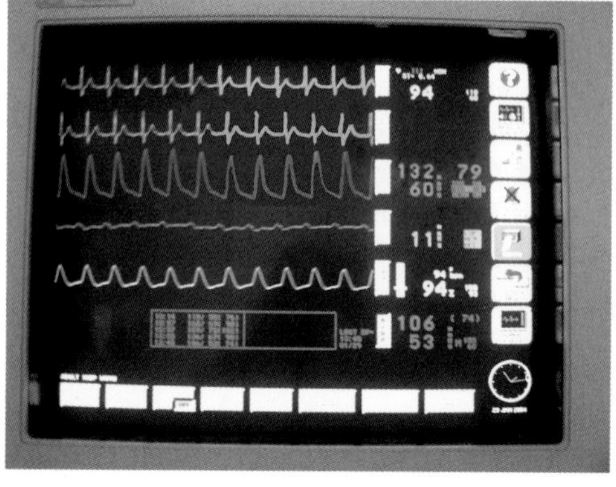

Figure 6.2 ICU monitor displaying ECG, invasive blood pressure and waveform, CVP and waveform, Sp_{O_2}.

Arterial blood pressure

In health, systemic arterial blood pressure is closely regulated to ensure adequate tissue perfusion. In critically ill patients, mean arterial pressure (MAP) should normally be maintained above a minimum value of 70 mmHg. However, it may be appropriate to aim for a higher value in elderly patients (as blood pressure tends to increase with age) and in patients with known hypertension. It is very helpful to know what is 'normal' for an individual patient, and such information may be available in the patient's case notes.

MAP is dependent on cardiac output (CO) and systemic vascular resistance (SVR) according to the formula: $MAP = CO \times SVR$ (analogous to Ohm's law). Measurement of arterial blood pressure is thus a relatively crude indicator of cardiac performance and circulatory flow, as it may be normal or elevated in the presence of a low cardiac output and poor tissue perfusion. Interpretation of the blood pressure must be taken in the context of other clinical measurements such as the state of the peripheral circulation, urine output, trends in acid–base balance, and serial lactate measurement. In critically ill patients it is often useful to measure cardiac output as well (see below).

Arterial blood pressure is usually monitored invasively on the ICU as it is more accurate and continuous. The presence of an indwelling arterial catheter allows blood sampling without the need for repeated puncturing of veins or arteries. The advantages and disadvantages of direct measurement are shown in Table 6.3. A catheter is inserted percutaneously into a suitable artery, ideally the radial artery of the non-dominant hand (common alternatives being the femoral and dorsalis pedis arteries, less commonly the brachial and axillary arteries). The arterial blood pressure is transmitted via saline-filled tubing to a pressure transducer that converts the mechanical signal to a very small electrical signal, proportional to the pressure. This signal is amplified and displayed on a monitor both as a waveform and as pressure readings: systolic, diastolic, and mean. Ensuring that the transducer is at the level of the heart and exposing it to the atmosphere when zeroing the monitor ensures accuracy of the system. To prevent the system becoming blocked, it is flushed constantly with heparinized saline at approximately 3 mL/h from a pressurized source to prevent backflow. Central venous and pulmonary artery pressures are measured using the same system.

Table 6.3 Advantages and disadvantages of direct arterial blood pressure measurement.

Advantages
- Accuracy (particularly at extremes of high and low pressure)
- Continuous measurement gives immediate warning of important changes in blood pressure
- Shape of arterial waveform gives information relating to myocardial contractility and other haemodynamic variables
- Facility for frequent arterial blood sampling

Disadvantages
- Requires expertise for insertion and subsequent care
- Potentially inaccurate if apparatus is not set up correctly
- Haematoma at puncture site
- Infection at puncture site/bacteraemia/septicaemia
- Disconnection haemorrhage
- Embolization
- Arterial thrombosis

Recently, specialized arterial catheters have become available that analyse the shape of the arterial waveform (pulse contour analysis) to determine stroke volume and hence cardiac output (see later).

Central venous pressure (CVP)

CVP is a surrogate index of the patient's circulating volume (or, more correctly, right ventricular preload). It is useful for directing fluid therapy in cases of dehydration, hypovolaemia due to haemorrhage and sepsis syndrome, and in the diagnosis and management of heart failure. Absolute values are often of less importance than following trends that occur in response to therapeutic interventions (e.g. fluid challenge) or during deterioration in a patient's condition. The routes commonly used to measure CVP are discussed in Chapter 3. Multilumen central venous catheters (CVCs) are generally used with 3–5 separate infusion channels. A CVC may also be used for a variety of other purposes in the ICU, as shown in Table 6.4.

Table 6.4 Uses and complications of central vein catheterization.

Uses
- Measurement of central venous pressure
- Infusion of:
  - irritant solutions, e.g. KCl
  - vasoconstrictor agents, e.g. noradrenaline, adrenaline, dopamine
  - parenteral nutrition
- Insertion of temporary cardiac pacing wire
- Insertion of pulmonary artery flotation catheter
- Venous access:
  - for haemodialysis, haemofiltration, plasmaphoresis, etc.
  - in the absence of peripheral veins
  - during cardiac arrest

Complications
- Arterial puncture/catheterization
- Haematoma
- Infection/septicaemia
- Pneumothorax (most likely with subclavian approach)
- Damage to adjacent structures
- Air embolism

There are two main limitations in monitoring CVP. First, although CVP is used to estimate circulating volume, it is a relatively crude index as quite large changes in volume can occur with relatively little change in CVP. This is because venous tone (and hence capacitance) varies in response to sympathetic outflow and infusion of vasopressor agents. Secondly, therapy is directed towards optimizing the filling pressures on the right side of the heart. While the filling pressures of the right and left sides are normally closely related, this relationship may not always be reliable in critically ill patients, particularly those with pre-existing cardiac or respiratory disease. In this situation, it may be of greater therapeutic value to monitor and optimize conditions for the left ventricle.

Pulmonary artery pressure

Pressures in the pulmonary artery are monitored using a pulmonary artery flotation catheter (PAFC), often referred to as a 'Swan–Ganz' catheter. This is a specialized multilumen catheter with an inflatable balloon and a temperature thermistor at its distal end.

A PAFC is inserted percutaneously usually via either the internal jugular or subclavian vein in the same manner as inserting a CVP line. Once the catheter is in a central vein, as indicated by the pressure waveform, the balloon is inflated. The forward flow of blood towards the heart carries the balloon so that the catheter can be advanced into and through the right atrium and ventricle until its tip lies in a main branch of the pulmonary artery (Fig. 6.3). In this position, an indirect assessment of the filling pressure in the left ventricle can be made. This is often referred to as the wedge pressure because the balloon is advanced until it 'wedges' in the pulmonary artery and the pressure is measured distal to the balloon. The wedge pressure is usually closely related to the left ventricular end-diastolic pressure. This is a more accurate indication of the preload to the left ventricle than the CVP. The wedge pressure is influenced by many of the factors affecting CVP, and trends are more useful than absolute values. Complications associated with PAFC insertion are listed in Table 6.5.

Table 6.5 Complications of pulmonary artery catheterization.

- All of the complications associated with central venous catheterization
- Ventricular dysrhythmias
- Pulmonary infarction
- Pulmonary artery rupture
- Knot formation
- Balloon rupture
- Subacute bacterial endocarditis
- Pericardial tamponade
- Damage to tricuspid or pulmonary valve

In addition to invasive pulmonary pressure data, a PAFC can also be used to measure cardiac output (utilizing the thermal dilution principle) and several derived haemodynamic variables (e.g. stroke volume, systemic and pulmonary vascular resistance, left ventricular stroke work). Mixed venous blood can be sampled from the pulmonary artery which, in conjunction with an arterial blood sample, is used to calculate the arteriovenous oxygen content difference. Fibreoptic PAFCs are also available that function according to the same spectrophotometric principle of the pulse oximeter and

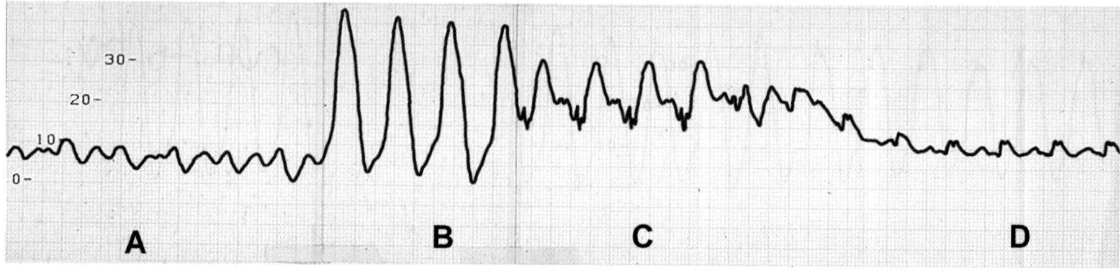

Figure 6.3 Pressure trace on insertion of a pulmonary artery catheter: (A) in the right atrium, (B) in the right ventricle, (C) in the pulmonary artery, (D) in the pulmonary artery with balloon inflated ('wedged').

provide continuous measurement of mixed venous oxygen saturation.

Oxygen delivery to the tissues and consumption by them can be calculated according to the following equations:

Oxygen delivery (mL/min) = cardiac output (L/min) × arterial oxygen content (mL/L); normal value ~1000 mL/min.

Oxygen consumption (mL/min) = cardiac output (L/min) × arteriovenous oxygen difference (mL/L); normal value ~250 mL/min.

Oxygen content blood (mL/L) = haemoglobin concentration (g/L) × oxygen saturation (expressed as a decimal fraction) × oxygen binding capacity of haemoglobin (1.34 mL/g); normal value ~200 mL/L.

Their routine use in patients has declined over recent years following the publication of several large studies not only questioning the benefit of such a general approach but also suggesting the possibility that any benefits might actually be outweighed by potential complications. The large, multicentre PAC-Man study from the UK published in 2005 finally concluded that there was evidence of neither benefit nor harm by managing all critically ill patients with a PAFC. Furthermore, the demise of invasive cardiac output monitoring has coincided with an expansion in the use of less invasive forms of cardiac output monitors (see below). Accordingly, many intensivists no longer insert PAFCs in critically ill patients as a matter of routine but reserve them for particular indications.

Non-invasive cardiac output monitors

The PAFC has always been considered to be a clinical gold standard for the measurement of cardiac output. Correct insertion requires expertise and is associated with a number of potentially life-threatening complications. A variety of non-invasive (or, perhaps more accurately, minimally invasive) cardiac output monitors have been introduced into clinical practice based on different physical and physiological principles and are now being used increasingly on the ICU.

Oesophageal doppler monitor (ODM)

Insertion of an ODM is relatively non-invasive, the ultrasound emitter–sensor being passed into the oesophagus, in a technique similar to that of inserting a nasogastric tube, to lie anterolateral to the descending aorta. The underlying principle is that flow through a cylinder (aorta) is proportional to the velocity of the fluid and the cross-sectional area of the tube. The cross-sectional area of the aorta is estimated using a nomogram based on the patient's age, weight, and height. The velocity of blood flow along the aorta is determined using the Doppler principle; ultrasound waves from the probe are reflected back from the moving bloodstream and the change in frequency monitored. Monitoring is continuous and allows acute changes in cardiac output to be detected (Fig. 6.4). The ODM is a useful tool, particularly for following trends in cardiac output following therapeutic interventions or during acute deterioration in a patient's condition. It has been shown to be particularly useful in guiding fluid replacement (targeted volume management) in patients undergoing major surgery where it had been shown to be associated with improved outcome and reduced length of hospital stay. Although it is easier to insert than a PAFC, there are potential sources of inaccuracy in the measurement of cardiac output; the descending aorta only receives a proportion of the cardiac output and the cross-sectional area of the aorta has to be estimated. Both of these are calculated automatically. Finally, for optimal results, the probe must be correctly aligned by the operator with the axial flow in the aorta using the displayed waveform.

Thoracic electrical bioimpedance (TEB)

In this technique, several electrodes are placed around the thoracic wall, and the electrical resistance of the thorax to a small high-frequency current (bioimpedance) is measured. TEB is inversely proportional to the fluid volume of the thorax, which varies throughout the cardiac cycle as the heart contracts and relaxes. An estimate of stroke volume can therefore be made from changes in thoracic bioimpedance. TEB is genuinely

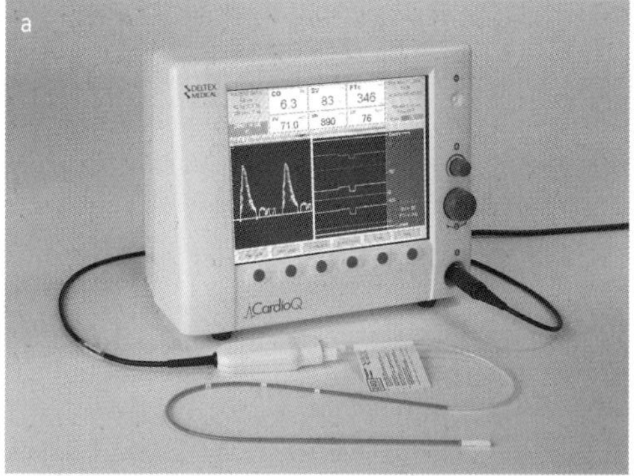

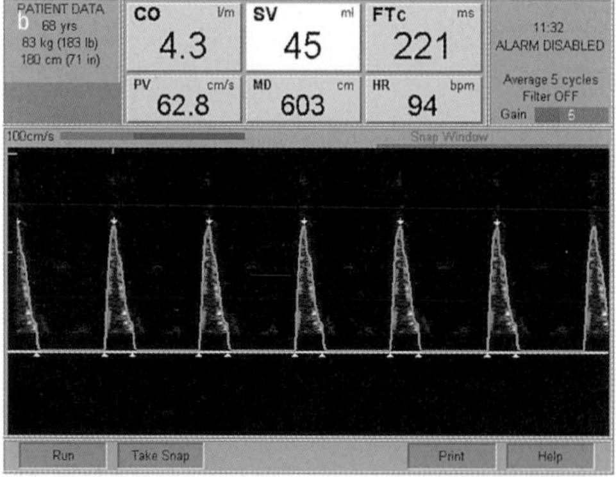

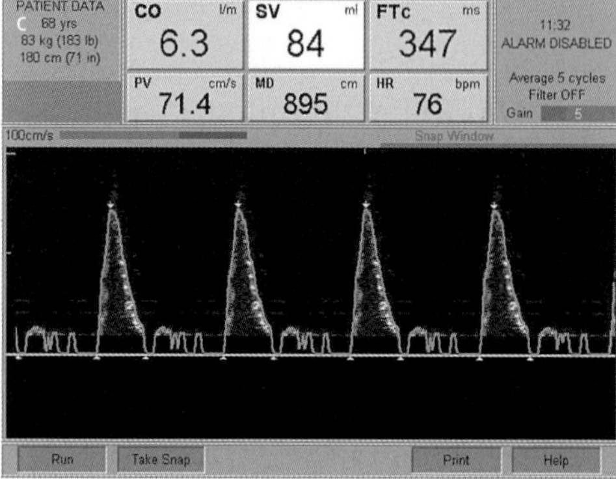

Figure 6.4 (a) Transoesophageal Doppler machine and oesophageal probe. (b) Narrow waveform, typical of hypovolaemia. (c) Broadening of the waveform after giving IV fluid.

non-invasive, depending as it does only on the attachment of surface skin electrodes. Measurements are, however, extremely sensitive to the precise positioning of the electrodes. Other causes of inaccuracy include irregular dysrhythmias and any acute changes in the water content of the thorax (e.g. pulmonary oedema, pleural effusion) which necessarily limit its utility in many critically ill patients.

Pulse contour analysis (PCA)

Pulse contour analysis hinges on the principle that the stroke volume of the left ventricle is proportional to the area under its pressure–time curve. The waveform obtained by an arterial catheter is analysed by the monitor, and changes in the waveform (pulse contour) reflect changes in stroke volume. As PCA does not measure either flow or volume directly, it needs to be calibrated using an alternative means of measurement of cardiac output. It tends to be more accurate when placed in a large proximal artery (e.g. femoral). An alternative approach developed from the above is the technique of arterial pulse power analysis (LiDCO™). This determines a nominal stroke volume which is then calibrated against an independent dye dilution measurement; a known amount of lithium chloride is injected and sensed by a lithium ion-selective electrode. Any arterial site can be used as the system reviews the power of the whole pulse contour, not just systolic area. It has been shown to correlate well with thermodilution methods for measuring cardiac output. Although these devices can be considered to be invasive in that an arterial catheter is required, it is likely that the large majority of patients in whom continuous cardiac output monitoring is indicated will need invasive blood pressure measurement.

Pulse oximetry

The pulse oximeter provides a simple, non-invasive, continuous assessment of the oxygenation of the peripheral tissues (SpO_2). It therefore gives a simultaneous indication of the degree of oxygenation of arterial blood by the respiratory system and the ability of the cardiovascular system to deliver it to the tissues. By providing continuous monitoring, it can be used to give an early warning of deterioration in a patient's condition. The principles of operation are described in Chapter 2.

Monitoring renal function

All patients on the ICU should have their plasma urea, creatinine, and electrolytes (Na, K, Ca, Mg, phosphate, etc.) measured at least once daily, and urine output monitored hourly (hence all patients are normally catheterized). The absolute minimum daily urine volume that will accommodate the normal urinary solute load (urea, sulphates, phosphates, and other waste products of metabolism) assuming that the kidneys are capable of maximally concentrating the urine (to 1400 mosm/L) is approximately 500 mL. If the kidneys are incapable of concentrating the urine maximally, the obligatory minimum daily urine production will need to be greater than this. Urine production below 500 mL/day is termed oliguria. In clinical practice, oliguria is also often defined as a rate of urine production less than 0.5 mL/kg/h. Anuria, when absolutely no urine is produced at all, is relatively uncommon. The possibility of a blocked urinary catheter should always be considered, and the catheter flushed or changed before concluding that the patient really is anuric.

Although renal failure may be diagnosed by observing oliguria/anuria and by raised serum urea and creatinine concentrations, this approach can be somewhat crude and limited. Renal failure may still be present with a normal or even raised urine output (polyuric renal failure). Plasma urea may be elevated in critically ill patients as a consequence of the increased protein catabolism that is a feature of the stress response, or by acute gastrointestinal haemorrhage (so-called protein meal). The relationship between renal glomerular filtration rate (GFR) and plasma creatinine concentration is not linear. The normal GFR of approximately 125 mL/min greatly exceeds homeostatic requirements. In fact, the GFR needs to fall below about 30–40 mL/min before there is any significant rise in plasma creatinine concentration above the normal reference range. This fact, of course, ensures that renal failure does not occur after a nephrectomy if the function of the preserved kidney is normal. Furthermore, as plasma creatinine levels are also related to muscle mass, elderly or cachetic patients with reduced muscle mass will tolerate a greater reduction in glomerular filtration before the plasma creatinine rises. Accordingly, estimation of the GFR is a much better approach to monitoring renal function in critically ill patients. As creatinine is freely filtered at the glomerulus and relatively little net creatinine is either added or removed from the glomerular filtrate by the processes of renal tubular secretion or reabsorption, creatinine clearance (the conceptual volume of blood from which all of the creatinine is completely removed by the kidneys each minute) is a good working approximation to the GFR:

$$\mathrm{GFR} = \mathrm{CR}_{\mathrm{CL}} = \frac{\text{rate of urinary production} \times \text{urine[Cr]}}{\text{plasma[Cr]}}$$

The rate of urine production may be calculated from a 24 h collection with a plasma creatinine estimation at the mid-point of the collection. In practice, many ICUs simply collect an overnight sample of urine (e.g. 0000–0800 h) and send it for assay together with that morning's plasma urea and electrolyte sample.

Neurological assessment

Neurological assessment of patients on the ICU is often difficult because of the use of sedatives and neuromuscular blocking drugs. Ideally, muscle relaxants should be avoided unless absolutely necessary. A minimal level of sedation should be employed, titrated for each individual and compatible with a comfortable, settled patient who is nonetheless easily rousable. This is often much easier said than achieved.

Scoring systems such as the Glasgow Coma Scale (GCS) and Ramsay sedation scale (see Table 6.6) can be used, provided that allowances are made for the effects of drugs and the presence of a tracheal tube. Patients who have undergone major intracranial surgery or sustained a severe acute brain injury may have their ICP monitored. A variety of devices are available that are placed via a small (burr) hole in the skull into the brain parenchyma, lateral ventricle, subarachnoid,

Table 6.6 Ramsay sedation scale.

Level	Conscious level
1	Restless and agitated
2	Cooperative, calm, orientated
3	Asleep, responds to verbal command
4	Asleep, responds briskly to glabellar tap
5	Asleep, responds sluggishly to glabellar tap
6	No response

subdural, or extradural space. ICP monitors utilize either a transducer whose electrical resistance changes with pressure (Codman ICP monitor) or a fibreoptic catheter in which changes in ICP alter the reflection of the light beam (Camino ICP monitor). The aim is to keep the ICP below 20 mmHg whilst maintaining cerebral perfusion pressure (MAP–ICP) above 70 mmHg. When patients are deeply sedated, and particularly if ICP monitoring is not available, it may be necessary to transport brain-injured patients for serial computed tomography (CT) scans to detect the development of raised ICP radiologically (e.g. cerebral oedema). This is always a major undertaking, and a risk–benefit analysis must always be undertaken first.

Monitoring hepatic function

Hepatic dysfunction may be primary or, more commonly in the context of critically ill patients, secondary to another disease process (Table 6.7). Liver function is monitored by serum bilirubin, albumin, transaminases (AST, ALT, GGT), alkaline phosphatase, prothrombin time (PT), and activated partial thromboplastin time (APTT). The PT is probably the most sensitive indicator of hepatic reserve and prognosis in severe liver failure. Although many critically ill patients develop biochemical hepatic dysfunction during the acute phase of their illness, in general this tends to recover as the patient recovers from the primary illness. However, mortality from acute fulminant hepatic failure in critically ill patients is almost universal, particularly if the patient has pre-existing liver disease, unless a liver transplant is performed.

Table 6.7 Causes of hepatic dysfunction.

Primary
- Viral hepatitis, A, B, C, cytomegalovirus, Epstein–Barr virus, etc.
- Alcoholic liver disease
- Drug-induced hepatitis: halothane, sodium valproate, isoniazid, paracetamol overdosage
- Autoimmune hepatitis/cirrhosis
- Acute fatty liver of pregnancy
- Inborn error of metabolism, e.g. Wilson's disease

Secondary
- Sepsis syndrome
- Hypoxia
- Hypotension
- Cardiac failure
- Cholestasis
- Cholangitis
- Total parenteral nutrition (TPN)

Miscellaneous

Routine haematology (haemoglobin concentration, white cell count, platelet count, etc.) should be assessed daily. Trace elements (e.g. Cu, Zn, Se) may need monitoring in patients resident on the ICU for longer than a few days, particularly those receiving parenteral nutrition.

Mechanical ventilation

One of the most common interventions on the ICU is mechanical ventilation of critically ill patients who have developed respiratory failure (often as a component of multiple organ failure) or when respiratory failure is thought to be imminent in an exhausted patient. Hypoxaemia ($PaO_2 < 8$ kPa) with or without accompanying hypercapnia ($PaCO_2 \geq 6.6$ kPa) is usually present despite high-flow oxygen therapy. The aim of mechanical ventilation is to optimize oxygenation of the patient and to allow a period of respite by relieving the patient of the work of breathing. The causes of respiratory failure are diverse (see Table 5.4). A common presentation in critically ill patients is acute respiratory distress syndrome (ARDS). Following a variety of insults, pulmonary capillaries become hyperpermeable, with leakage of fluid and the development of non-cardiogenic pulmonary oedema. This results in areas of ventilation/perfusion mismatch, severe hypoxaemia, tachypnoea, and, eventually, physical exhaustion as the patient tries to compensate.

During mechanical ventilation, the physiological negative pressure phase of spontaneous inspiration is replaced by a positive pressure phase in which respiratory gas is driven into the lungs by the ventilator. As a result, the distribution of gas flow through the lungs, the shape of the chest wall, and the pattern and extent of diaphragmatic movement are altered. Although this may lead to a small increase in ventilation/perfusion mismatching, the net result is usually beneficial in improving arterial PaO_2 and $PaCO_2$ values. The reasons for this include:

- reliable administration of up to 100% O_2;
- reduced oxygen consumption by a sedated, ventilated patient;
- ventilation with larger tidal volumes than can be achieved by the dyspnoeic patient breathing spontaneously;
- application of PEEP.

The latter two measures increase the FRC of the lungs above a critical level (the closing volume). This reduces the extent of collapse of small airways, thus improving ventilation/perfusion matching.

Positive pressure ventilation may also relieve a failing left ventricle and alleviate cardiogenic pulmonary oedema by reducing venous return to the heart during inspiration as the intrathoracic pressure rises. The abnormally high left ventricular preload accompanying left ventricular failure is reduced and the overstretched muscle fibres are able to return to a more optimal size for efficient contraction. Mechanical ventilation may also reduce left ventricular afterload as it produces a positive pressure gradient between the thoracic and abdominal aorta during inspiration. Although the gradient is relatively small, the reduction in work required of the left ventricle may be significant. The work of breathing is also reduced, and alveoli flooded with oedema fluid are opened.

Critically ill patients requiring ventilation often have a reduction in lung compliance (stiffer lungs) and an increase in resistance to respiratory gas flow. Consequently, ICU ventilators are programmed with a wide variety of settings to optimize ventilation and gas exchange (Fig. 6.5). They allow the intensivist a great deal of control over the pattern of inspiratory gas flow and adjustment of the time taken for inspiration and expiration, usually expressed as the inspiratory to expiratory (I:E) ratio. Furthermore, different ventilation modes are available which allow patients' spontaneous but inadequate respiratory efforts to be assisted, such as pressure support ventilation (PSV) and synchronized intermittent mandatory ventilation (SIMV).

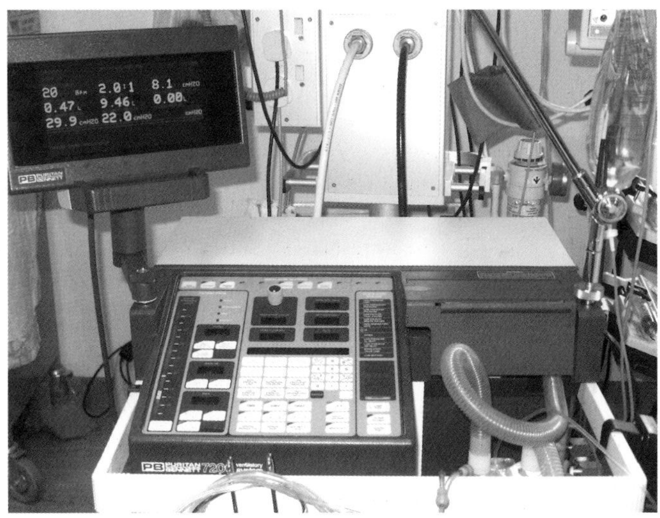

Figure 6.5 ICU ventilator. Soft keys allow control of ventilator settings with display of volumes and pressures generated.

Intubation and tracheostomy

The majority of patients on the ICU are ventilated during the acute stage of their illness through a cuffed tracheal tube inserted via the mouth or, less commonly, via the nose. The cuff should have a large volume to minimize the pressure exerted on the tracheal mucosa (high-volume, low-pressure cuff). A tracheal tube is very uncomfortable, and patients usually require sedation and analgesia to tolerate its presence. Tracheal intubation is also associated with difficult oral hygiene, infection, and ulceration. These factors become a more significant problem during the period of recovery when attempts are being made to wean the patient off ventilatory support, as it now becomes necessary to reduce the level of sedation and analgesia to facilitate this process. Furthermore, it is well known that the continued presence of a tracheal tube is associated with a higher incidence of long-term complications, particularly tracheal stenosis. Accordingly, if the period of tracheal intubation is longer than about a week, it is usual to perform a tracheostomy.

Until 20 years or so ago, this necessitated a formal surgical procedure in the operating theatre, usually by an ENT surgeon. However, most tracheostomies are now performed using a percutaneous technique on the ICU by intensivists using purpose-designed kits. In the most popular method, a tapered dilator is passed along a guidewire through a small incision, until the track is large enough to accommodate the tracheostomy tube (Fig. 6.6). Percutaneous tracheostomy is simple and quick to perform (usually less than half an hour), and is associated with a very low incidence of complications. Consequently, it is increasingly performed relatively soon after the patient's admission to the ICU, particularly when it is anticipated that weaning of the patient may be delayed or difficult.

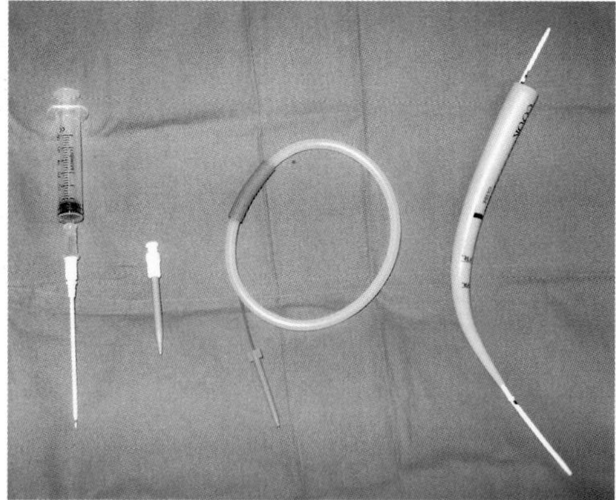

Figure 6.6 Percutaneous tracheostomy kit showing needle for initial puncture, Seldinger wire, and tapered dilator.

Non-invasive positive pressure ventilation

Although most critically ill patients admitted to the ICU will be ventilated via a tracheal tube, non-invasive positive pressure ventilation (NIPPV) is being used increasingly as the evidence supporting its efficacy has grown (Fig. 6.7).

NIPPV is not a replacement for IPPV, rather it is a complementary therapeutic approach. It has advantages and disadvantages when compared with IPPV (Table 6.8). On the face of it, NIPPV is preferable to IPPV:

- the patient remains conscious;
- a tracheal tube is not required;
- ICU admission is not mandatory;
- the patient continues to breath spontaneously throughout (albeit with positive pressure assistance);
- successful weaning is usually more straightforward;
- the risk of ventilator-associated pneumonia (VAP) is reduced.

However, many patients are simply too ill, either to tolerate the procedure or to provide the necessary cooperation and spontaneous respiratory effort required. The airway is not protected during NIPPV and the risk of pulmonary aspiration is ever present in patients with a reduced GCS (<8) or who are too weak to mount an effective cough.

In general, there are two broad groups of patients in whom NIPPV may be considered: patients whose physical status and acute illness does not preclude progression to ICU admission and IPPV should NIPPV fail; and patients for whom ICU admission is considered to be inappropriate and NIPPV represents the limit of treatment.

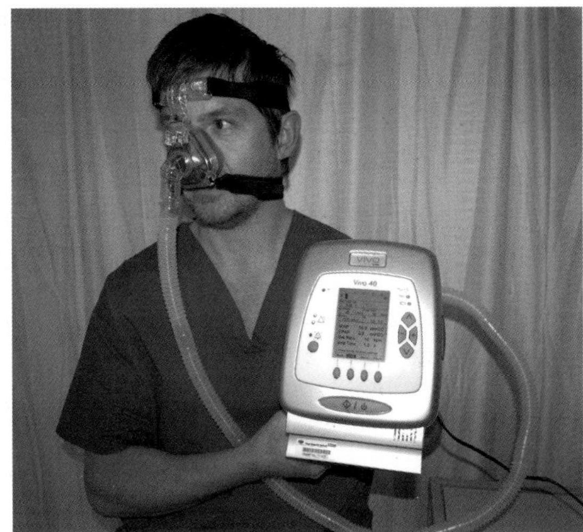

Figure 6.7 Demonstration of NIPPV equipment. Volunteer wearing a tight-fitting nasal mask and holding the ventilator. This generates a positive pressure to augment the volume of spontaneous breaths. Peak inspiratory and expiratory pressures, inspiratory rate and time can be adjusted according to need.

The largest group of patients in whom the efficacy of NIPPV has been studied is those with acute exacerbation of COPD. Several large randomized controlled trials have convincingly demonstrated improvements in respiratory acidosis and hypoxaemia, and a reduction in length of hospital stay, morbidity, and mortality. A significant proportion of these patients will improve without recourse to IPPV. The benefits are clearer in more severe exacerbations (pH <7.3, $PaCO_2$ >45 mmHg). There is now a clear consensus that such patients should generally be treated with NPPV before considering ICU admission and IPPV. Markers of successful treatment include younger age, unimpaired level of consciousness, and a prompt positive response within the first few hours.

Patients with acute cardiogenic pulmonary oedema may also benefit from NIPPV. The

Table 6.8 Comparison of IPPV and NPPV.

IPPV	NPPV
• ICU admission required	• May be managed in a variety of specialized areas
• Tracheal intubation or tracheostomy required	• Administered using a tight-fitting face or nasal mask
• Protects the airway against pulmonary aspiration	• No airway protection afforded
• Sedation/anaesthesia required	• Sedation not required (nor desirable)
• Does not require any patient cooperation	• Patient must be cooperative enough to tolerate the procedure
• Does not require any respiratory effort from the patient	• Patient must be capable of breathing spontaneously
• Abolition of normal feeding and speech	• Feeding and speech retained
• High levels of inspiratory pressure and PEEP may be provided	• Inspiratory pressure and PEEP more limited
• Reduces patients' oxygen requirements significantly	• More limited reduction in patients' oxygen requirements
• Diagnostic/therapeutic bronchoscopy through tracheal tube facilitated	• Patient may be too ill to tolerate bronchoscopy
• Increased risk of ventilator-associated pneumonia (VAP)	• Less risk of VAP
• Difficulties of successfully weaning patient off ventilatory support and sedation as they have been conscious and breathing spontaneously throughout	• Sedation not an issue and respiratory weaning potentially easier

potential advantageous effects of positive pressure ventilation on the failing heart have already been described. There is good evidence that simple application of CPAP as an adjuvant to inotropic and other pharmacological therapies reduces myocardial oxygen demand and improves oxygenation and cardiac output. The evidence for the greater efficacy of NIPPV over CPAP in acute cardiogenic pulmonary oedema is less convincing than is the case in acute exacerbation of COPD. Some studies actually suggest an increase in the rate of MI and death in patients treated with NIPPV rather than CPAP, especially in the presence of respiratory acidosis.

Sedation and analgesia

Critically ill patients require varying degrees of sedation and analgesia. These two terms are not synonymous. Anxiety, agitation, and pain may exist separately or in combination. They have different aetiologies and require different drugs and techniques. Mechanically ventilated, intubated patients are often deeply sedated during the early acute phase of critical illness. As their condition stabilizes and improves, consideration is then given to weaning them off sedation. Patients often become confused and disorientated by their illness during this period as their level of consciousness rises, and are likely to become agitated by their environment. Disruption of the normal awake–sleep cycle, alarms constantly sounding off, difficulties in communication, and performance of a variety of procedures (physiotherapy, suction down the tracheal tube or tracheostomy, insertion of intravascular catheters) may all trigger anxiety and/or pain. For patients with insight, the realization of the seriousness of their condition and the contemplation of their own mortality can be frightening. Confused, agitated patients are a risk to themselves as they may inadvertently pull out tracheal tubes, nasogastric tubes, or intravascular catheters. Heart rate, arterial blood pressure, myocardial work, and oxygen demand are all needlessly elevated with accompanying risks. The psychological trauma engendered may also hinder recovery. An appropriate level of sedation produces calm, cooperative patients who are thus easier to nurse and treat. On the other hand, patients admitted to the ICU following major surgery or trauma will suffer if good analgesia is not provided. Many of the invasive procedures that are undertaken on patients are painful and, as mentioned above, even the presence of the tracheal tube itself can be distressingly uncomfortable.

Until relatively recently, it was common practice to paralyse and deeply sedate all patients so that they were completely unaware of their surroundings until they were deemed 'recovered' from their critical illness. It is now realized that such deep sedation is not only unnecessary, but may also be harmful (Table 6.9). A minimum level of sedation and analgesia is now advocated, with a daily period of cessation of the sedative and analgesic drugs in most patients (sedation holiday) to allow a better assessment of the depth of sedation and prevent accumulation of drugs that may take days to wear off.

The ideal level of sedation is one in which the patient is calm, awake, or rousable to voice/light touch and orientated during appropriate periods of the day. The Ramsay sedation scale (Table 6.6) is one of a number of sedation scales in common use, a score of 2–4 being considered satisfactory depending on the clinical situation and time of day. Before ascribing agitation to inadequate sedation or analgesia, it is important to exclude and treat physiological derangements such as hypoxia, hypercapnia, hypotension, and any metabolic derangements.

The most commonly used sedative drugs are midazolam and propofol. The latter is less likely to accumulate when given by continuous infusion over several days, but is more likely to cause or exacerbate systemic hypotension in septic patients.

Table 6.9 Problems associated with deep sedation.

- Immunosuppression
- Increased incidence of infection
- Prolonged recovery time
- Impaired function of the gastrointestinal tract
- Loss of contact with reality, with an adverse effect on psychological well-being

Table 6.10 Potential indications for continuous infusion of a muscle relaxant and potential problems with their use.

Indication	Effect of paralysis
• Poor lung/chest wall compliance and associated high inflation pressure • Acute severe brain injury • High metabolic demand in severe sepsis, burns, MH, etc.	• Improved compliance, reduced inflation pressure • Prevention of acute damaging surges in intracranial pressure in response to coughing, straining, agitation, etc.
Problems associated with muscle relaxants	
• Inability to assess level of sedation/conscious level • Awareness in a paralysed patient • Critical illness myopathy	

Opioids such as morphine, fentanyl, alfentanil, and remifentanil are used when analgesia is required. Morphine and fentanyl may accumulate when given by prolonged infusion. This is less of a problem with alfentanil. Remifentanil is ultrashort acting, even when given by prolonged infusion, its effects wearing off within minutes of cessation. Remifentanil is often useful when intense analgesia is required for a painful procedure (e.g. during a percutaneous tracheostomy) or in situations when it is necessary to sedate a patient for a relatively short period of time. For example, a patient admitted to the ICU unconscious after a severe head injury may need to be deeply sedated and ventilated for a period of 24–48 h. If this is achieved using a combination of propofol and remifentanil, it is usually possible to assess higher neurological function without the confounding variable of residual sedation within a very short time of cessation. Sedative and analgesic drugs are usually given together as the combination tends to work synergistically—the effect of the two drugs together is greater than the simple additive effect that might be anticipated. This allows smaller doses to be administered with less accumulation and fewer side-effects.

Regional anaesthetic techniques are also used, particularly continuous epidural analgesia using a combination of a low concentration of local anaesthetic and opioid (see Chapter 4). This technique is suitable for pain relief following surgery or trauma to the thorax, abdomen, pelvis, and lower limbs. It is often easier to wean patients off mechanical ventilation more quickly in the presence of epidural analgesia as they can take deep breaths and cough forcefully, uninhibited by pain or the respiratory depressant effects of systemic opioids.

Muscle relaxants were used almost routinely in mechanically ventilated intubated patients 20 years or so ago, but are now reserved for selected critically ill patients only, as problems associated with their use have become apparent. In particular, critical illness myopathy is a serious complication of prolonged use of muscle relaxants. Neuromuscular blockade functionally denervates skeletal muscle, the result of which is to accelerate and potentiate muscle wasting that is already occurring because of disuse atrophy. The patient develops profound global weakness (it often appears that the patient is still paralysed!), and weaning from ventilatory support is delayed, as is further onward progress of the patient. The relatively few indications for continuous infusion of muscle relaxants and associated problems are summarized in Table 6.10.

Nutrition

Maintenance of adequate nutrition is an essential element of the care of critically ill patients. Sufficient calories must be provided to fuel the acute stress response in which basal metabolic rate is usually elevated. Protein must be provided to minimize catabolism of skeletal muscle. Vitamins, essential amino and fatty acids, trace elements, and other nutrients are all necessary, particularly when nutritional support is required for more than a few days. The support and advice of a dietician, experienced in the special requirements of critically ill patients, is very helpful, and ideally all patients on the ICU will be reviewed on a daily basis.

Where possible, patients should be fed enterally, and there is no reason why feeding cannot be commenced on day one in many patients. *If the gut is working, use it!* Enteral feeding is simpler to administer, less expensive, more physiological, and associated with fewer complications than total parenteral nutrition (TPN). The presence of food within the gut stimulates intestinal blood flow and facilitates earlier recovery of normal gastrointestinal function. It also protects the gastric and upper small intestinal mucosa from developing acute peptic ulceration. Enteral nutrition is commonly administered through a nasogastric tube. Increasingly, a feeding jejunostomy is performed when the patient has presented with a surgical problem requiring laparotomy as enteral feeding is likely to be established more quickly—often the rate-limiting step in absorbing enteral nutrition is gastric emptying rather than function of the small intestine. If there is a delay in establishing enteral nutrition, or it is contraindicated, TPN should be commenced. Indications for TPN and associated complications are listed in Table 6.11.

Table 6.11 Indication for total parenteral nutrition and associated complications.

Indications

- Ileus following major bowel surgery, MOFS, deep sedation
- Acute pancreatitis
- Inflammatory bowel disease
- Short bowel syndromes
- Malabsorption syndromes
- Multiple organ failure
- Severe catabolic states, e.g. extensive burns, severe sepsis, major trauma

Complications

- Central line sepsis
- Acute gastric erosion
- Hyperglycaemia
- Specific mineral or vitamin deficiencies
- Less satisfactory nutrition of the luminal mucosa of the gut
- Hepatic dysfunction
- Expensive

Critically ill patients are at risk of developing acute erosion and ulceration of the gastric mucosa, particularly those who are unable to tolerate enteral feeding when the action of gastric acid is unopposed. The most appropriate method of ulcer prophylaxis is provision of enteral nutrition at the earliest opportunity. Inhibition of gastric acid production itself (e.g. with ranitidine or a proton pump inhibitor such as pantoprazole) provides prophylaxis against acute gastric ulceration when enteral feeding is not possible. However, abolishing the acid environment of the stomach also risks causing bacterial overgrowth in the upper gastrointestinal tract that may increase the risk of so-called VAP.

Infection control

Hospital-acquired (nosocomial) infections are common on the ICU and are associated with increased morbidity and mortality. They are increasingly due to multiply antibiotic-resistant organisms such as methicillin-resistant *Staphylococcus aureus* (MRSA). Critically ill patients on the ICU have a number of risk factors for developing infection (Table 6.12). Common infections involve the lower respiratory tract in ventilated patients (VAP), septicaemia associated with intravenous and arterial lines, and surgical wound infections. Prevention of nosocomial infection should be a priority (Table 6.13). The single most important aspect of prevention is the practice of good hygiene standards.

Table 6.12 Risk factors for nosocomial infection on the ICU.

- Extremes of age
- Pre-existing medical conditions
- Poor nutritional status
- Immunosuppressive effect of illness, drugs
- ICU is a breeding site for antibiotic-resistant strains of bacteria
- Breach of body surface defences:
- Tracheal intubation
- Urinary catheter
- IV and arterial lines
- Raised intragastric pH due to H_2 antagonists

Table 6.13 Prevention of nosocomial infection on the ICU.

Good basic hygiene standards
• Scrupulous washing of hands immediately before and after contact with patient; routine wearing of gloves and aprons
• Regular disinfection of ventilator tubing or use of disposable equipment
• Use of bacterial/viral filters between patient and ventilator
• Insertion of IV lines, catheters under full asepsis
• Regular toileting of patient, particularly surgical wounds and sites of insertion of IV lines, catheters
• High index of suspicion for intravascular catheter sepsis and removal/change of lines in patients with new or worsening features of sepsis
Optimize nutritional status of patient
Avoid overuse of 'prophylactic' broad-spectrum antibiotics

Supporting the failing organ

Respiratory failure

The causes of respiratory failure and the principles of mechanical ventilation have already been discussed. The most important therapy is oxygen—a life-saving 'drug'. It must be administered in sufficient concentration to raise the PaO_2 to a minimum acceptable level, approximately 10.5 kPa (80 mmHg), although lower levels may be well tolerated in patients with chronic hypoxia. All severely hypoxic patients should be given as high an inspired oxygen concentration as possible, by facemask initially. Unfortunately, as described earlier, many patients are denied high-flow oxygen therapy, due to unwarranted concern that their respiration is dependent on a hypoxic drive. Only a minority of patients with *severe* chronic obstructive airways disease (classically described as blue bloaters) are dependent on a hypoxic ventilatory drive, and these patients should have their oxygen therapy carefully titrated. It is not that unusual to find hypoxic patients without any previous history of chronic obstructive airways disease receiving 28% oxygen because of such fears, and the authors have even seen young, fit patients admitted with acute severe asthma being denied 100% oxygen. It is important to remember that it is the partial pressure of oxygen in arterial blood (PaO_2) that is responsible for respiratory drive, *not* the inspired oxygen concentration. If there are serious concerns regarding a severely hypoxic patient with chronic respiratory disease and a suspected hypoxic ventilatory drive, immediate referral to an expert is advised.

Although pulmonary oxygen toxicity may occur when oxygen is administered in a concentration >40% for a prolonged period, it is both illogical and dangerous to withhold higher concentrations in hypoxic patients with severe respiratory failure because of such fears. In any case, oxygen toxicity is more closely correlated with PaO_2 than inspired oxygen concentration.

The majority of patients admitted to the ICU require mechanical ventilation. Many of these have ARDS and require the use of higher inflation pressures to provide an adequate tidal volume. In ARDS, the lungs become very stiff (decreased compliance) due to alveolar and interstitial oedema, acute inflammatory infiltrates, atelectasis, and pulmonary fibrosis. Although it is obvious that these patients would die without mechanical ventilation, in recent years it has become increasingly apparent that mechanical ventilation itself may further injure the lung in critically ill patients. This lung damage is caused by:

- high inflation pressures (barotrauma);
- overdistension of more compliant areas of the lung (volutrauma);
- repeated 'snapping' open and closed of collapsed alveoli during inspiration and expiration (atelectrauma).

There is now good evidence that limiting the plateau inflation pressure below a maximum of 30 cmH_2O and accepting lower tidal volumes (e.g. 6 mL/kg rather than 10–12 mL/kg) may reduce ICU length of stay and mortality. Application of a high PEEP (approximately 10–15 cmH_2O) also helps to minimize alveolar collapse and atelectrauma. This 'protective ventilatory strategy', using a combination of a specialized mode of ventilation called pressure-controlled ventilation (PCV), a reversed I:E ratio, and high PEEP, has become common in the UK and elsewhere. It is recommended in the Surviving Sepsis Campaign guidelines (see later). One of the consequences of protective ventilation is an increased $PaCO_2$ and respiratory acidosis—permissive hypercapnia. However, this is well tolerated by most critically ill patients, although the consequent rise in ICP dictates that hypercapnia should not be permitted in patients with acute severe brain injury.

In general, VAP is common in critically ill patients and correlates with the length of time that a patient requires invasive mechanical ventilation. Managing the patient in the semirecumbent position (head of the bed raised to 45°) has been shown to reduce the incidence of VAP.

Appropriate antibiotics should be given in the presence of a chest infection. It is essential to obtain a specimen of sputum for microbiological examination and antibiotic-sensitivity testing, ideally from the *lower* respiratory tract. Bronchodilators may be useful in patients with bronchospasm associated with asthma or chronic obstructive airways disease, chest infection, pulmonary aspiration, or ARDS. Bronchodilators are commonly administered as a nebulized mist directly to the respiratory tract (e.g. salbutamol, ipratropium). They may also be given by IV infusion (salbutamol, adrenaline, aminophylline), although there is a greater risk of dysrhythmias. Effective physiotherapy is an essential part of respiratory care for all patients on the ICU. Techniques used by physiotherapists in helping to expectorate secretions from the lungs include the positioning of patients to facilitate postural drainage of secretions and percussion of the chest to help loosen secretions. Suctioning of the trachea and upper airways is important as nearly all critically ill patients, whether sedated and paralysed or not, are incapable of coughing effectively because of generalized muscle weakness.

There are two other techniques practised on some ICUs in severe respiratory failure and ARDS.

Pulmonary arterial vasodilator therapy (inhaled nitric oxide (NO) gas or nebulized prostacyclin)

The rationale for vasodilator therapy is that the inhaled drug is delivered only to well-ventilated alveoli where it is a potent pulmonary arterial vasodilator. Pulmonary arterioles associated with poorly ventilated alveoli remain unaffected. It may be anticipated that this will lead to an improvement in the ventilation/perfusion ratio and, in practice, the initial response of the patient is often a significant improvement in oxygenation. However, the results of clinical trials have been disappointing and there are as yet insufficient data to demonstrate a beneficial effect on mortality from ARDS. Pulmonary artery vasodilatation therapy has rather fallen out of fashion in recent years.

Prone ventilation of patients

The potential benefits of this technique are derived from the fact that prolonged adoption of the supine posture leads to collapse of dependent (posterior) areas of the lung, increasing ventilation/perfusion mismatch. Reversing the posture facilitates re-expansion of the dependent lung. Prone ventilation does appear to improve oxygenation temporarily. Unfortunately, the further benefits of pronation remain unproven, particularly a reduction in mortality. Turning patients prone is potentially hazardous and may result in accidental extubation of the patient, withdrawal of CVP and arterial lines, and pressure damage affecting particularly the eyes and face. However, when undertaken by teams of doctors and nurses experienced in the procedure, the risk of complications is low. Although some ICUs have a low threshold for pronating patients where it is seen as an almost routine aspect of the management of patients with ARDS, it is more common to reserve its use for those patients whose oxygenation is unsatisfactory despite a high inflation pressure and/or high inspired oxygen concentration.

Cardiovascular failure

The principles of treatment of cardiovascular failure are to optimize:

- conditions for the left ventricle in order to achieve an appropriate preload, stroke volume, cardiac output, and hence oxygen delivery to the tissues;

• the state of the circulatory system so that the cardiac output is distributed to vital organs at sufficient pressure for capillary beds to be well perfused.

In clinical practice, these principles are followed by:

• *Correcting hypovolaemia with fluid challenges* Increasing left ventricular preload so that it is functioning at the peak of the Frank–Starling curve. This first step is the single most important prerequisite for optimal cardiovascular performance.

• *Treating dysrhythmias adversely affecting cardiac performance* The most common on the ICU is atrial fibrillation, and this sometimes resolves spontaneously when the patient is adequately fluid resuscitated. IV amiodarone is the most effective drug used to treat atrial fibrillation in critically ill patients, and acts either by reducing the ventricular response rate or by pharmacological cardioversion back into sinus rhythm.

• *Improving myocardial contractility* An inotropic agent (e.g. dobutamine) may be required to increase cardiac output to a satisfactory level. Cardiac output may be monitored using a PAFC, oesophageal Doppler ultrasound probe, or arterial pulse wave contour analysis.

In severe sepsis syndrome, MAP is often inadequate in spite of a normal or even elevated cardiac output. In this situation, a vasopressor (a drug that vasoconstricts systemic arterioles) is necessary, for example noradrenaline. Vasodilators are only occasionally useful on the ICU to 'offload' a failing left ventricle. The majority of patients who benefit from these drugs have usually suffered an MI. They are not usually mechanically ventilated and are admitted to the CCU rather than the ICU.

The use of inotropes and vasopressors mandates invasive monitoring of the cardiovascular system to direct therapy.

What targets should be aimed for with respect to MAP and cardiac output in critically ill patients with multiple organ failure?

Useful indicators include the state of the peripheral circulation (cold and shut down or warm and well perfused), trends in acid–base balance, and urine output (although urine output is of little use in the context of acute renal failure). Lactic acid is produced by anaerobic metabolism, and trends in serum lactate concentration can provide useful information on whether or not oxygen delivery to the tissues and oxygen consumption by the tissues is adequate.

It is usually appropriate to aim for a MAP of at least 70 mmHg. However, elderly patients and patients with pre-existing hypertension may require a significantly higher arterial pressure. On the other hand, younger patients may tolerate a lower pressure. Defining a satisfactory cardiac output in critical illness is more problematic. It is known that oxygen requirements are elevated during critical illness. Thus, values of cardiac output within the 'normal range' may be inadequate. However, following evidence that driving the cardiovascular system towards 'supranormal goals' did not improve mortality and could even increase it, most intensivists now adopt a more conservative approach. An indirect, evidence-based approach that can be applied to any patient with a CVC is measurement of the oxygen saturation of central venous blood ($S_{CV}O_2$).

In health, arterial oxygen saturation is approximately 97% and mixed venous oxygen saturation approximately 75%—the tissues extract approximately 25% of the 1000 mL of oxygen delivered to them per minute. Measurement of $S_{CV}O_2$ is therefore a useful indicator of the adequacy of cardiac output. If cardiac output is insufficient, the tissues will extract more oxygen from the blood as it flows through them and the $S_{CV}O_2$ will fall. It has been shown that maintaining $S_{CV}O_2$ at >70% correlates with reduced mortality. This may be achieved by appropriate fluid loading, use of inotropic therapy (e.g. dobutamine), and transfusion of red blood cells. Although a haemoglobin concentration of 70–80 g/L is well tolerated in most critically ill patients, in the context of an $S_{CV}O_2$ <70% it is appropriate to transfuse red blood cells above this low threshold in order to increase the oxygen-carrying capacity of the blood.

Acute renal failure

Acute renal failure is a common problem in critically ill patients. Although there are many causes of renal failure (Table 6.14), in the critically ill patient it usually results from failure to maintain an adequate renal perfusion pressure (prerenal failure) due, for example, to hypovolaemia. The kidneys attempt to maintain blood pressure and circulating volume by producing a minimal volume and maximal concentration of urine. However, once urine production falls below approximately 500 mL/day, the kidneys are unable to excrete all the waste products of metabolism, with the result that uraemia, metabolic acidosis, and hyperkalaemia develop.

If the reduction in renal perfusion and oxygenation is severe enough, not only does urine production stop but the kidneys also become ischaemic. Severe widespread necrosis may then ensue, mainly affecting the tubules (acute tubular necrosis, ATN), culminating in oliguria or anuria. Once ATN has developed, even restoration of a satisfactory blood pressure and circulating volume will not lead to immediate restoration of urine production. However, if the patient is appropriately resuscitated, there is a good chance that renal function will eventually recover as the patient recovers, although there is often a delay of 2–3 weeks before urine production restarts. When it does, it is typically high-output, low-concentration in nature, when particular attention needs to be paid to fluid and electrolyte balance. Pending recovery, the patient will require renal replacement therapy (see below).

Table 6.14 Aetiology of acute renal failure.

Prerenal
- Dehydration, e.g. vomiting, diarrhoea
- Haemorrhage
- Cardiogenic shock
- 'Third space losses', e.g. trauma, major surgery, bowel obstruction, etc.

Renal
- Acute tubular necrosis (usually secondary to severe prerenal failure)
- Sepsis
- Severe obstructive jaundice
- Blood transfusion reaction
- Myoglobinaemia secondary to ischaemic muscle damage and rhabdomyolysis
- Peritonitis

'Medical' causes
- Acute pyelonephritis
- Acute glomerulonephritis
- Acute pancreatitis
- Nephrotic syndrome
- Bowel obstruction
- Vasculitis
- Burns
- Renal vein thrombosis

Postrenal
- Bilateral obstruction to renal outflow (e.g. tumour)

Although prerenal factors are commonly implicated in acute renal failure affecting critically ill patients, some patients may already have pre-existing intrinsic chronic renal failure due to other causes. The two may present together (acute on chronic renal failure). The distinction between prerenal and intrinsic renal failure may be aided by biochemical investigations (Table 6.15).

Table 6.15 Differentiation of prerenal from intrinsic renal failure.

Index	Prerenal	Intrinsic renal
Urine concentration	High Specific gravity ≥1020 Osmolarity >550 mosmol/L	Dilute Specific gravity 1010 Osmolarity <350 mosmol/L
Urine (Na)	<20 mmol/L	>40 mmol/L
Urine/plasma osmolar ratio	≥2 : 1	1.1 : 1
Urine/plasma [urea]	≥20 : 1	<10 : 1
Urine/plasma [creatinine]	≥40 : 1	<10 : 1
Plasma urea (mmol/L)/creatinine (μmol/L) ratio	>0.1	<0.1

An inherently unstable cardiovascular system, the need for continued infusion of large volumes of fluid to combat the extravasation of circulating volume through leaky capillaries, and the use of potent inotropic and vasopressor drugs mean that these patients are often unable to tolerate the rapid fluid and ionic shifts associated with intermittent haemodialysis techniques, which may precipitate cardiovascular collapse. Peritoneal dialysis is also of limited value in the ICU as it does not have the capacity to maintain homeostasis in hypermetabolic patients or remove fluid rapidly enough when required. In addition, it is often not possible in patients after abdominal surgery and in those with abdominal sepsis.

Therefore, continuous haemofiltration (a process analogous to the filtration that occurs naturally in the glomeruli of the kidneys) is more often used as the preferred method of renal support on the ICU. An extracorporeal circulation is set up, containing a filter with an artificial semipermeable membrane. Although flow through the filter may be driven by the patient's own arterial pressure (continuous arteriovenous haemofiltration, CAVH), it is more usual to employ venovenous haemofiltration (CVVH) driven by a mechanical roller pump (Fig. 6.8). In addition, modern equipment permits the use of combination therapy in which both haemofiltration and dialysis occur simultaneously (CVVHD). The maximum creatinine clearance obtained is much less than that during haemodialysis. Consequently, CVVH must be run continuously in contrast to the short (several hours) intermittent (2–3 times per week) episodes of standard haemodialysis. However, as alluded to above, this disadvantage is also an advantage in that it promotes haemodynamic stability.

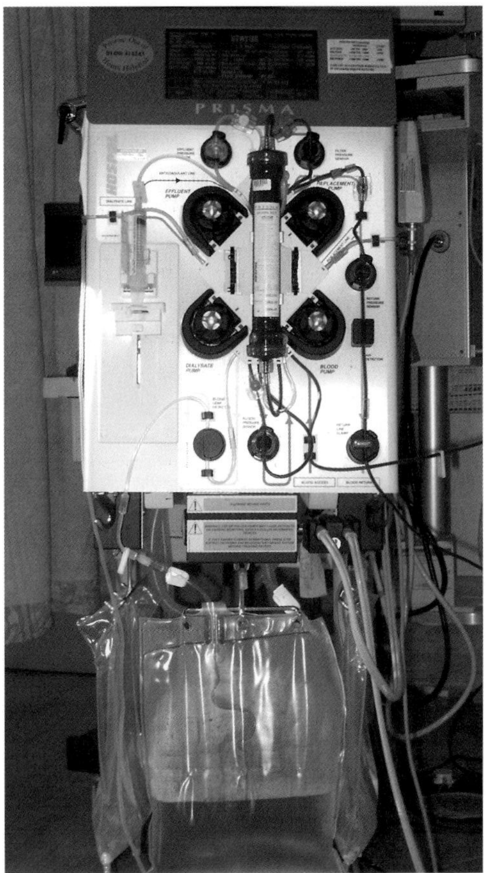

Figure 6.8 CVVH equipment. The vertical, central structure is the filter/dialysis membrane. There are four pumps: the one at the bottom right pumps blood in from a central vein into the filter; that at the bottom left pumps fresh dialysate fluid into the filter; the top left pumps out effluent from the filter (consisting of dialysate fluid plus ultrafiltrate); and the top right pump delivers replacement fluid to the patient to maintain fluid balance.

Sepsis syndrome, septic shock, systemic inflammatory response syndrome (SIRS), and multiple organ failure syndrome (MOFS)

Although there is considerable overlap between these conditions, they describe different pathophysiological conditions.

• *Sepsis syndrome and septic shock* Sepsis is a condition in which the host is overwhelmed by an infecting organism which proliferates in the bloodstream (septicaemia) and is therefore often diagnosed on blood culture. Septic shock is the presence of circulatory shock (low arterial blood pressure, organ hypoperfusion, and inadequate oxygen delivery to the tissues) caused by septicaemia. Many of the adverse circulatory effects observed in sepsis are due to endotoxins and

Table 6.16 The systemic inflammatory response syndrome.

Defined as the presence of two or more of the following:
• Temperature >38°C or <36°C
• Heart rate >90 beats/min
• Tachypnoea >20 breaths/min or $PaCO_2$ <32 mmHg
• White blood cell count >12 × 10^9/L, or <4 × 10^9/L, or >10% immature forms

exotoxins. Endotoxin is a complex of the lipopolysaccharide component of the cell membrane of Gram-negative organisms, whereas exotoxin is a soluble chemical secreted by microorganisms, including bacteria, fungi, and protozoa, into the circulation. Previously, Gram-negative organisms caused the majority of infections in critically ill patients. However, patterns of infection in the ICU have changed over recent years, reflecting the admission of ever older and sicker patients, the increasing use of invasive techniques, and the widespread use of broad-spectrum antibiotics. Thus, a shift towards more infections caused by Gram-positive bacteria and fungi has been observed. A worrying development has been the increasing prevalence of strains with multiple antibiotic resistance such as MRSA.

• *SIRS* This the clinical manifestations of the hypermetabolic, inflammatory state seen after any major insult to the body, and is defined in Table 6.16. The insult may be infection, in which case SIRS and sepsis syndrome describe the same pathophysiology. However, infection is not the only trigger for SIRS, and other causes include major trauma, burns, and acute pancreatitis.

The clinical features of sepsis syndrome and SIRS are similar, with hypermetabolism, inflammation, and circulatory shock due to systemic vasodilatation and extravasation of fluid (via leaky capillaries). In the lungs, these manifestations present as ARDS. Elsewhere, oxygen delivery to cells is compromised by shunting of blood away from capillary beds through arteriovenous channels that open in response to the inflammatory changes. Oxygen consumption by cells may also be reduced as a consequence of intracellular dysfunction of the mitochondria. The result of all these derangements is lactic acidosis due to oxygen supply–demand imbalance, the development of an oxygen debt, and an increase in anaerobic metabolism.

Like any other inflammatory response, SIRS is a physiological mechanism for defence of the body after a major insult, facilitating eradication of infection and tissue repair. The problem is that the host response becomes amplified and uncontrolled, contributing to further tissue damage and organ dysfunction.

• *Multiple organ failure syndrome* The failure of two or more organ systems (respiratory, cardiovascular, renal, gastrointestinal, haematological, hepatic, neurological) requiring therapeutic intervention and support, usually caused by sepsis and/or SIRS. The evidence base underpinning the recommended approaches to the management of critically ill septic patients with actual or potential multiple organ failure has been published under the aegis of the Surviving Sepsis Campaign. These guidelines describe a diverse range of diagnostic and therapeutic interventions summarized in Table 6.17. A full discussion of these guidelines is outside the scope of this book. However, some key points relating to immediate resuscitation that should be accomplished within the first 6 h are outlined below.

Early diagnosis of sepsis is essential. An indicative history and/or findings on clinical examination suggestive of the diagnosis should lead to appropriate further investigations to confirm the diagnosis and, wherever possible, localize the primary focus of infection. SIRS will be present in a majority of cases. A full microbiological screen should be performed as soon as possible, including blood cultures, and broad-spectrum antibiotics then administered. It may be necessary for the patient to undergo emergency surgery once adequately resuscitated if the cause of sepsis is surgical.

Any patient with suspected sepsis who satisfies the criteria for SIRS should be considered at risk for the development of septic shock and multiple organ failure, particularly if MAP <65 mmHg or a lactic acidosis is present. The serum lactate level should therefore be determined as soon as possible. Lactic acidosis develops when oxygen demand is not met by oxygen supply and metabolism

Table 6.17 Summary of Surviving Sepsis Campaign guidelines for the management of critically ill septic patients.

- Initial resuscitation (to be accomplished within the first 6 h of presentation)
  - Serum lactate measurement
  - Blood cultures taken before administration of broad-spectrum antibiotics
  - Administer antibiotics within 3 h of presentation to the emergency department
  - Deliver an initial bolus of fluid of = 20 mL/kg if mean arterial pressure <65 mmHg or serum lactate concentration >4 mmol/L with further boluses according to response
  - Start a vasopressor (e.g. noradrenaline) via a central line if patient does not respond to fluid challenges
  - Achieve and maintain central venous pressure >11 cmH_2O
  - Achieve and maintain central venous oxygen saturation ($S_{CV}O_2$) >70%
- Diagnosis
- Antibiotics
- Source control
- Fluid therapy
- Vasopressors
- Inotropic therapy
- Steroids
- Activated protein C
- Blood products
- Mechanical ventilation
- Sedation, analgesia, and neuromuscular blockers
- Glucose control
- Renal replacement
- Bicarbonate therapy
- Deep venous thrombosis prophylaxis
- Stress ulcer prophylaxis
- Consideration of limitation of support

becomes anaerobic. Inadequate oxygen supply is multifactorial, and causes include inadequate oxygenation of arterial blood, inadequate cardiac output, inadequate tissue perfusion pressure, and failure of the cardiac output to reach the cells (arteriovenous shunting). Furthermore, the tissues may fail to utilize delivered oxygen (histotoxic hypoxia—due to the presence of bacterial toxins and endogenous inflammatory mediators). Lactic acidosis may precede the development of systemic hypotension and so is a useful early indicator of trouble.

As ever, an ABC approach is essential. If arterial oxygenation is unsatisfactory, appropriate measures must be taken immediately to rectify the situation. This will always include the administration of high-flow oxygen using a facemask with attached reservoir bag, and may require the patient to be anaesthetized to permit tracheal intubation and mechanical ventilation. An initial rapid fluid bolus of at least 20 mL/kg should be given, repeated as necessary according to response. There is no clear evidence of the superiority of crystalloids (e.g. normal saline, Hartmann's solution) versus gelatin- or starch-based colloids (e.g. Haemaccel, voluven) in this situation, and either may be used.

If the condition of the patient remains unsatisfactory as determined by serial measurement of MAP and serum lactate, the patient should be transferred to a high dependency area if not already there, and arterial catheters and CVCs inserted. The utility of the CVC is three-fold: it permits measurement of CVP, administration of a vasopressor agent such as noradrenaline, and measurement of $S_{CV}O_2$. A CVP = 11 cmH_2O should be achieved and maintained by administration of fluid. If MAP fails to reach the target level, a vasopressor should be introduced. A vasopressor is a drug with predominantly alpha-adrenergic (vasoconstrictor) effects which tends to oppose the profound vasodilatation seen in septic shock. They are potent agents with short plasma half-lives and must therefore be administered via a syringe pump. Invasive monitoring of arterial blood pressure with an arterial line is mandatory when using vasopressors as it is essential that blood pressure is measured continuously and accurately. A significant proportion of critically ill patients have shock refractory to treatment with both fluids and vasopressors. Such patients often have sepsis-induced adrenal suppression. Although corticosteroids do not exhibit their own intrinsic vasopressor activity, they do exert a permissive effect on the vasopressor activity of catecholamines such as noradrenaline. Accordingly, it is recommended that steroids are administered in cases of refractory shock (e.g. hydrocortisone 300 mg per day).

Once these goals have been achieved, a sample of blood is taken from the CVC and the saturation measured. The target level is $S_{CV}O_2$ >70%. If the level is lower than this, oxygen delivery is inadequate for tissue requirements and the oxygen extraction ratio ((arterial oxygen content – venous oxygen content)/arterial oxygen content) has increased significantly above the normal of 0.25. Attempts should be made to increase oxygen delivery by transfusion of red blood cells if the haematocrit is lower than normal and by administration of an inotropic agent with predominantly beta-adrenergic effects (e.g. dobutamine), in an attempt to increase myocardial contractility, stroke volume, and cardiac output.

Further reading

The Acute Respiratory Distress Syndrome Network. Ventilation with lower tidal volumes as compared with traditional tidal volumes for acute lung injury and the acute respiratory distress syndrome. *New England Journal of Medicine* 2000; **342**: 1301–8.

Bernard GR, Vincent JL, Laterre PF *et al.*, and the Recombinant human protein C Worldwide Evaluation in Severe Sepsis (PROWESS) study group. Efficacy and safety of recombinant human activated protein C for severe sepsis. *New England Journal of Medicine* 2001; **344**: 699–709.

Boldt J. Clinical review: hemodynamic monitoring in the intensive care unit. *Critical Care* 2002; **6**: 52–9.

Caples SM, Gay PC. Noninvasive positive pressure ventilation in the intensive care unit: a concise review. *Critical Care Medicine* 2005; **33**: 2651–8.

Cuthbertson BH, Smith GB. Editorial: a warning on early-warning scores! *British Journal of Anaesthesia* 2007; **98**: 704–6.

Dellinger RP, Carlet JM, Masur H *et al.* Surviving Sepsis Campaign guidelines for management of severe sepsis and septic shock. *Critical Care Medicine* 2004; **32**: 858–73.

Esmonde L, McDonnell A, Ball C *et al.* Investigating the effectiveness of critical care outreach services: a systematic review. *Intensive Care Medicine* 2006; **32**: 1713–21.

Galley HF. *Critical care focus 1: renal failure.* London: BMJ Books, 1999.

Galley HF. *Critical care focus 2: respiratory failure.* London: BMJ Books, 1999.

Galley HF. *Critical care focus 5: antibiotic resistance and infection control.* London: BMJ Books, 2001.

Gao H, McDonnell A, Harrison DA *et al.* Systematic review and evaluation of physiological track and trigger warning systems for identifying at-risk patients on the ward. *Intensive Care Medicine* 2007; **33**: 667–79.

Gattinoni L, Tognoni G, Pesenti A *et al.* Effect of prone positioning on the survival of patients with acute respiratory failure. *New England Journal of Medicine* 2001; **345**: 568–73.

Harvey S, Harrison DA, Singer M *et al.* Assessment of the clinical effectiveness of pulmonary artery catheters in management of patients in intensive care (PAC-Man): a randomised controlled trial. *The Lancet* 2005; **366**: 472–7.

Hodgetts TJ, Kenward G, Vlackonikolis I *et al.* Incidence, location and reasons for avoidable in-hospital cardiac arrest in a district general hospital. *Resuscitation* 2002; **54**: 115–23.

Lightowler JV, Wedzicha JA, Elliott MW. Non-invasive positive pressure ventilation to treat respiratory failure resulting from exacerbations of chronic obstructive pulmonary disease: Cochrane systematic review and meta-analysis. *British Medical Journal* 2003; **326**: 185.

McQuillan P, Pilkington S, Allan A *et al.* Confidential inquiry into quality of care before admission to intensive care. *British Medical Journal* 1998; **316**: 1853–8.

Meduri GU, Headley AS, Golden E *et al.* Effect of prolonged methylprednisolone therapy in unresolving acute respiratory distress syndrome. *Journal of the American Medical Association* 1998; **280**: 159–65.

NHS Estates. *Facilities for critical care.* Health Building Note 57. London: The Stationery Office, 2003.

Nolan J, Baskett P, Gabbott D *et al.* *Advanced life support provider course manual*, 4th edn. London: Resuscitation Council (UK), 2000.

Oh TE. *Intensive care manual*, 5th edn. London: Butterworths, 2003.

Rivers E, Nguyen B, Havstad S *et al*. Early Goal-Directed Therapy Collaborative Group. Early goal-directed therapy in the treatment of severe sepsis and septic shock. *New England Journal of Medicine* 2001; **345**: 1368–77.

Smith GB, Osgood VM, Crane S. ALERT: a multiprofessional training course in the care of the acutely ill adult patient. *Resuscitation* 2002; **52**: 281–6.

Surviving Sepsis Campaign evidence-based reviews. *Critical Care Medicine* 2004; 32 (11): Supplement.

Van den Berghe G, Wouters P, Weekers F *et al*. Intensive insulin therapy in the critically ill patients. *New England Journal of Medicine* 2001; **345**: 1359–67.

Useful websites

http://www.dh.gov.uk/en/Publicationsandstatistics/Publications/PublicationsPolicyAndGuidance/DH_4006585

[Department of Health (UK). Comprehensive Critical Care. A review of adult critical care services. May 2000.]

http://www.dh.gov.uk/en/Publicationsandstatistics/Publications/PublicationsPolicyAndGuidance/DH_4121049

[Department of Health (UK). Quality Critical Care. Beyond 'Comprehensive Critical Care'. September 2005.]

http://www.ics.ac.uk/

[The Intensive Care Society (ICS). The publication section contains current UK national guidance on all aspects of critical care.]

http://www.sccm.org/

[This site contains current guidelines from the Society of Critical Care Medicine (SCCM) and reflects North American practice.]

http://www.ccmtutorials.com/

[Excellent, up-to-date interactive critical care tutorials.]

http://www.americanheart.org/presenter.jhtml?identifier=9181

[The American Heart Association scientific-statements section has numerous up-to-date guidelines.]

http://www.dh.gov.uk/en/Publicationsandstatistics/Publications/PublicationsPolicyAndGuidance/DH_4091873

[Department of Health (UK). Critical Care Outreach 2003: progress in developing services. This report contains guidance on best practice in this area.]

http://www.dh.gov.uk/en/Publicationsandstatistics/Publications/PublicationsPolicyAndGuidance/DH_072769

[Produced by the Critical Care Stakeholders Forum and National outreach Forum. Describes the role of Outreach services and provides quality indicators.]

http://www.brit-thoracic.org.uk/Portals/0/Clinical%20Information/NIV/Guidelines/NIV.pdf

[Guidelines on non-invasive ventilation in acute respiratory failure. British Thoracic Society Standards of Care Committee. *Thorax* 2002; 57: 192–211.]

http://www.pacep.org/

[Pulmonary artery catheter resource with haemodynamic monitoring tutorials. Free to use once registered.]

http://www.sfar.org/s/article.php3?id_article=60

[This site has information on all the various scoring systems used in critically ill patients, including on-line calculators.]

http://www.dicm.co.uk/papers.htm

[This is a personal website aimed at those taking the Diploma in Intensive Care Medicine Exam. It claims to list the top 100 critical care references and succeeds in most areas.]

http://www.ardsnet.org/

[The ARDS clinical network site. This contains updates on ARDS studies performed by the network.]

http://www.survivingsepsis.org

[Homepage of the Surviving Sepsis Campaign.]

http://www.ihi.org/IHI/Topics/CriticalCare/Sepsis/

[The Institute for Health Improvement website. This contains a huge amount of information on the management of severe sepsis including a description of so-called care bundles.]

All websites last accessed April 2008.

Self-assessment

6.1 Describe the principles of intra-arterial measurement of blood pressure. What are the advantages and disadvantages of this technique?

6.2 Give five common indications for inserting a central venous catheter in an ICU patient. Give four complications of this procedure.

6.3 Give five factors that put ICU patients at risk of nosocomial infection. What can be done to prevent nosocomial infections on the ICU?

6.4 What criteria are necessary to make a diagnosis of SIRS? List the key interventions that should be undertaken within the first six hours to resuscitate septic patients according to the Surviving Sepsis Campaign guidelines.

6.5 What are the common indications for mechanical ventilation on the ICU? How might IPPV improve gas exchange?

6.6 Patients with which chronic disease have been shown to benefit from non-invasive positive pressure ventilation (NPPV) and within this group who benefit the most? What are the potential advantages and disadvantages?

Answers to self-assessment questions

1. Anaesthetic Assessment and preparation for surgery

1.1. (*see pages 4–5*)
(a) By assessing activities of daily living: get dressed, distance walked on the flat, stairs climbed, run for a bus.
(b) By estimating how many METs the patient is capable of: jog, play squash (≥7 METs), gardening, walk on the flat (5–7 METS), symptoms when dressing (≤2 METs).
(c) Perform cardiopulmonary exercise testing: measure the patient's anaerobic threshold. If >14 ml/kg/min, no specific risk; <11 ml/kg/min high risk, ITU needed postoperatively.

1.2. (*see pages 7–8*)
(a) Look at the patient's oro-facial and cervical anatomy.
(b) Mallampati criteria.
(c) Thyromental distance.
(d) Wilson score.
(e) Calder test.

1.3. (*see page 11*)
I A healthy patient.
II A patient with a mild to moderate systemic disease process that does not limit the patient's activities in any way.
III A patient with severe systemic disease from any cause that imposes a definite functional limitation on activity.
IV A patient with a severe systemic disease that is a constant threat to life.
V A moribund patient unlikely to survive 24 h with or without surgery.
The patient described would be ASA III; she has systemic illnesses which impose a restriction on her functional activity, but they are not a constant threat to her life at present.

1.4. (*see pages 7–9*)
This is major surgery, according to the NICE guidelines she will need to have:
A full blood count (FBC) to identify: anaemic (low Hb) and its possible cause (MCV), occult infection (raised WCC), blood clotting problems (low platelet count).
Renal function tests (also called urea and electrolytes, U&Es): to identify electrolyte disturbances or impaired renal function as a result of her age, or as a consequence of treatment for hypertension (diuretics, ACEi).
ECG: to identify cardiac ischaemia, conduction disturbance or arrhythmia, and left ventricular hypertrophy.
In addition she will need:
Pulmonary function tests to assess the severity of her COPD.
If dyspnoeic at rest, cyanosed or has a FEV1 < 60% predicted, she will need arterial blood gases doing.
She will not need a chest x-ray as this is only required when there are signs or symptoms of

pulmonary disease and the patient is to undergo thoracic surgery.

2. The principles of anaesthesia

2.1. (*see page 29*)
An LED emits red light, alternating between two different wavelengths in the visible and infrared regions of the electromagnetic spectrum. These are transmitted through and absorbed by the tissues, oxyhaemoglobin, and deoxyhaemoglobin. The light reaching the photodetector is converted to an electrical signal. Absorption by the tissues is constant while absorption by blood varies with the cardiac cycle, allowing peripheral arterial oxygen saturation (Spo2) to be calculated.
Limitations:
It is unreliable; when there is severe vasoconstriction, with certain haemoglobins and when there is excessive movement of the patient.
It is affected by extraneous light.
It does not give any indication of the adequacy of alveolar ventilation.

2.2. (*see pages 20–21*)
Oxygen is stored in a vacuum-insulated evaporator at -180 degrees Celcius, and at 10–12 bar. The liquid vapourises and by the time it reaches the operating theatre it is a gas at ambient temperature.

Nitrous oxide is stored in a bank of cylinders, it is liquid at a pressure of 54 bar. Medical air is supplied either from cylinders or by a compressor.

All gases are distributed by the piped medical gas and vacuum system and reach the operating theatre at a pressure of 4 bar (medical gas also delivered at 7 bar to power instruments).

For safety, the hoses are colour coded (oxygen white, nitrous oxide blue and air yellow). They attach to the wall outlets via gas-specific probes and to the anaesthetic machines via non-interchangeable nut and union.

2.3. (*see pages 38–39*)
Suxamethonium molecules enter the neuromuscular junction and compete with Ach, binding to the postsynaptic (nicotinic) receptors on the motor end plate on the muscle membrane.

Muscle fasciculation is seen as the muscle membrane is depolarised.

This is followed by paralysis as the suxamethonium molecules remain bound to the receptors keeping the muscle membrane depolarised.

Recovery occurs spontaneously as suxamethonium is hydrolysed by the enzyme plasma (pseudo-) cholinesterase.

Normal neuromuscular transmission is restored after 4–6mins.

Side-effects:
Malignant hyperpyrexia.
Increased intraocular pressure.
Muscular pain.
Histamine release.
Prolonged apnoea in patients with pseudocholinesterase deficiency.
A significant rise in serum potassium in certain conditions.

2.4. (*see pages 43–44*)
They inhibit the enzyme cyclo-oxygenase (COX). This prevents the synthesis of inflammatory mediators (prostaglandins, prostacyclins and thromboxane A2) from arachidonic acids. There are two main isoenzymes of cyclo-oxygenase, COX-1, COX-2. The inhibition of COX-1 produces the unwanted effects, inhibition of COX-2 the desired therapeutic effects.

Relative contraindications	Absolute contraindications
High risk of intraoperative bleeding e.g. vascular surgery	Pre-existing renal dysfunction, hyperkalaemia
Concurrent use of ACE inhibitors, anticoagulants, nephrotoxic drugs	Cardiac failure
Hepatic dysfunction	Severe hepatic dysfunction
Bleeding disorders	History of GI bleeding
Elderly (>65 years)	Hypersensitivity to NSAIDs
Pregnancy and during lactation	Aspirin induced asthma
Asthma	

2.5. (*see pages 45–47*)

A stimulus of sufficient intensity triggers opening of (voltage-gated) sodium channels. Cell membrane potential increases from –70 mV to +20 mV (action potential). Adjacent voltage-gated sodium channels open, propagating the action potential along the nerve. In myelinated nerves action potentials can 'jump' between nodes of Ranvier to speed up conduction. The membrane is rapidly repolarised by loss of potassium ions (K+) from within the cell, and by active pumping out of Na+ in exchange for K+ by the Na/K pump.

Local anaesthetic drugs work by blocking the sodium channels from within the nerve cell, preventing entry of sodium and subsequent depolarization so that no action potentials can be initiated or propagated.

The relationship between concentration, volume, and dose is given by the formula:

Concentration (%) × Volume (ml) × 10 = dose (mg), therefore

$$0.75\% \times 15 \times 10 = 112.5 \text{ mg}$$

Toxic dose = 3 mg/kg, max 200 mg without adrenaline
6 mg/kg, max 500 mg with adrenaline

3. The practice of anaesthesia

3.1. (*see page 55*)

Advantages include:

Avoids repeated attempts at venepuncture in patients with poor veins.

Avoids venepuncture in an uncooperative child, or patients with needle phobia.

In patients with airway compromise, preserves spontaneous ventilation and if airway patency is threatened, further uptake of anaesthetic is prevented, limiting the problem.

Disadvantages include:

Unconsciousness occurs more slowly than with an IV drug.

Inhalational drugs are unpleasant to breathe.

Hypotension and a fall in cardiac output occur with increasing concentrations. This may be difficult to treat until IV access is obtained.

Hypercapnia (due to respiratory depression) and the vasodilator effect of these drugs lead to increased cerebral blood flow, making this technique unsuitable in patients with raised intracranial pressure.

3.2. (*see pages 61–62*)

Gold standard:

Measuring carbon dioxide in expired gas (capnometry).

Next best:

Use an oesophageal detector device.

Seeing the tracheal tube passing between the vocal cords.

Fogging on clear plastic tube connectors during expiration.

Less reliable signs are:

Breath sounds on auscultation.

Chest movement on ventilation.

Gurgling sounds over the epigastrium.

Decrease in oxygen saturation (late).

Complications:

Unrecognized oesophageal intubation.

Failed intubation and inability to ventilate the patient.

Failed ventilation after intubation.

Aspiration of regurgitated gastric contents.

Direct trauma to all structures from lips to lungs.

Trauma to adjacent structures during the procedure.

Hypertension and arrhythmias.

Vomiting.

Laryngeal spasm.

3.3. (*see page 66*)

Infusions of propofol to keep the patient unconscious and an opioid for analgesia (remifentanil, alfentanil). Boluses of fentanyl could also be used or alternatively a regional technique (epidural). A neuromuscular blocking drug will be required for muscle relaxation and ventilation with oxygen-enriched air.

Advantages:

Avoid potential toxic effects of inhalational anaesthetics and use of nitrous oxide

Improved quality of recovery.
Beneficial in certain types of surgery (neurosurgery)
Reduces pollution
Disadvantages:
Reliable IV access required.
Risk of awareness if IV infusion fails.
Cost of electronic infusion pumps.
Hypotension.

3.4. (*see pages 66–67*)
Indications:
When neuromuscular blocking drugs are used to facilitate surgical access, e.g. laparotomy.
During thoracotomy to prevent paradoxical movement.
To prevent unacceptable degree of respiratory depression.
To allow control of carbon dioxide and cerebral blood flow during neurosurgery.
Whenever a patient needs tracheal intubation for more than a few minutes e.g. prone surgery, full stomach, shared airway (ENT).
Potential adverse effects:
There is an increase in ventilation/perfusion (V/Q) mismatch, requiring the use of an increased inspired oxygen concentration.
Reduced venous return to the heart and cardiac output.
Hyperventilation and hypoventilation causing a respiratory alkalosis and a respiratory acidosis respectively with the associated effects on the oxyhaemoglobin dissociation curve.
Excessive tidal volume may cause lung injury.
Reduced systemic and pulmonary blood flow.

3.5. (*see pages 67–68*)
Avoids the systemic effects of drugs used for GA.
Respiratory depressant drugs avoided.
There is generally less disturbance of the control of coexisting systemic disease.
The airway reflexes are preserved.
May improve surgical access e.g. during laparotomy.
Reduced blood loss.
Can be continued postoperatively to provide pain relief.
Reduces complications after major surgery.
A reduction in the equipment required and the cost of anaesthesia.

3.6. (*see pages 79–80*)
Factors predisposing to regurgitation and aspiration:
A full stomach.
Gastric distension following face mask ventilation.
Delayed gastric emptying from any cause (e.g. trauma).
Obstetric patients.
Gastro-oesophageal reflux, hiatus hernia.
Obesity.
Prevention:
Reduction of residual gastric volume.
Increase pH of gastric contents.
Use of cricoid pressure.

3.7. (*see page 83*)
Clinical signs:
Severe hypotension.
Severe bronchospasm.
Widespread flushing.
Hypoxaemia.
Urticaria.
Angioedema, which may involve the airway.
Pruritus, nausea and vomiting.
Immediate management:
Stop all drugs, call for help.
Maintain a patent airway, give 100% oxygen.
Elevate the patient's legs.
Give adrenaline, boluses of 0.5 mL of 1:10,000 under ECG control. If no ECG available, give 0.5 mL of 1:1000 IM.
Ensure adequate ventilation.
Start a rapid intravenous infusion of crystalloids 10–20 mL/kg.
In the absence of a major pulse, start cardiopulmonary resuscitation.
Monitor: ECG, SpO_2, blood pressure, end-tidal CO_2, check the blood gases.

4. Postanaesthesia care

4.1. (*see pages 88, 91*)
Hypoventilation: airway obstruction (tongue), respiratory depression (drugs), mechanical

impairment (obesity), pulmonary dysfunction (smoking).
Ventilation/perfusion mismatch; reduced FRC (pain, obesity, elderly, upper GI surgery).
Diffusion hypoxia; use of nitrous oxide.

Oxygen masks:
Hudson; MC mask; 25%–60%. Flow dependent
Hudson with reservoir; up to 85%
Nasal catheter; 25–40%
Venturi masks; 24–60% depending on which used

4.2. (*see pages 92–93*)
Hypovolaemia; blood loss, inadequate fluid replacement.
Cardiac dysfunction; ischaemic heart disease, arrhythmia, valvular heart disease.
Vasodilatation; sepsis, extensive spread of epidural anaesthesia, anaphylaxis.

Management:
Ensure adequate oxygenation and ventilation.
Give intravenous fluid bolus and observe response.
Get help.
Stop external haemorrhage with direct pressure, get surgical assistance if internal haemorrhage suspected.
Cross-match blood.
Monitoring central venous pressure (CVP).
Treat any arrhythmias (check U&Es, ABGs).
Check extent of epidural action.
May need vasopressors and/or inotropes.

4.3. (*see pages 98–99*)
He will require a minimum of:
- Maintenance fluid, 1.5 ml/kg/hr water, 1.5 mmol/kg sodium and 1 mmol/l potassium:
  $1.5 \times 80 \times 24 = 2880$ ml water, 120 mmol sodium, 80 mmol potassium.
- In addition, he has signs of hypovolaemia (tachycardia, hypotension, oliguria and feels thirsty), probably as a result of third space losses. This will require an additional 1000 ml fluid (normal saline or Hartmann's).
- The losses from the drain will need replacing, 400 ml (saline or Hartmann's).
- He is hypokalaemic and hence will need extra potassium (40 mmol).
- He is anaemic and will require blood to raise his Hb to 9 g/dl.

Predicted total requirement:
4280 ml, 340 mmol sodium, 120 mmol potassium, 3 units of packed red blood cells.

There are a number of combinations of fluids that could be used. One regime that could be used to achieved this:
1 l 0.9% saline plus 40 mmol KCl over 4 hours.
1 l 0.9% saline plus 40 mmol KCl over 4 hours.
1 l 4% glucose/0.18% saline plus 20 mmol KCl over 6 hours.
1 l 4% glucose/0.18% saline plus 20 mmol KCl over 6 hours.
0.5 l 4% glucose/0.18% saline over 4 hours.
3 units PRBC concurrently.

The patient must be reviewed after 6–8 hours to see if there is any change in his status. Early consideration should be given to monitoring of his CVP.

4.4. (*see pages 102–103*)
A PCA device is a microprocessor-controlled syringe pump that can be programmed to deliver a predetermined dose of a drug intravenously and activated by the patient depressing a switch. The maximum dose in any period and any background infusion is predetermined to prevent overdose and after a dose has been delivered subsequent doses cannot be given for a preset period, the 'lockout period'. PCAs record the number of attempts made by the patient to access analgesia, allowing the dose to be adjusted to meet their requirements.
Advantages:
Analgesia matched to the patient's perception of the pain.
Reduced workload for the nursing staff.
Elimination of painful IM injections.
Greater certainty of adequate plasma levels.
Disadvantages:
Expensive to purchase and maintain.
Needs patient to understand how to use the PCA and be able to trigger the device.
Potential for overdose if incorrectly programmed.

4.5. *(see page 105)*
Hypotension. Treat acutely with IV fluid and vasopressors. Check the extent of the block; if extensive, reduce the rate of infusion.
Respiratory depression. Treat by supporting ventilation if necessary; stop the epidural infusion; give naloxone according to the severity; seek expert help.
Sedation. Treat by stopping the infusion; if unresponsive or the level of sedation progresses, give naloxone in 0.1 mg increments intravenously; seek expert help.
Pruritus. May respond to antihistamines, atropine or naloxone.
Retention of urine. May require short-term catheterization.

5. Recognition and management of the acutely ill patient on the ward

5.1. *(see pages 110–111)*
Look for: Paradoxical chest and abdominal movements, use of the accessory muscles of respiration, tracheal tug, intercostal recession
Feel for: Movement of air at the patient's mouth
Listen for: breath sounds at the mouth or nose. Noisy breathing means obstruction.

Management:
Head tilt, chin lift, suction – reassess.
Oropharyngeal or nasopharyngeal airway – reassess.
Give high flow oxygen.
If no improvement, urgent call for help, prepare for use of advanced airway.
If satisfactory, move on to assess adequacy of breathing.

5.2. *(see pages 113–114)*
Shock is the inadequate perfusion of the vital organs with oxygenated blood.

Assessment:
Look at the colour of the hands and digits, the state of the peripheral veins, level of consciousness, oliguria, signs of blood or extracellular fluid loss.
Feel limb temperature, measure the capillary refill time (CRT). Assess the peripheral pulses for; rate, volume, regularity/rhythm.
Listen to the heart sounds. A 3rd heart sound is indicative of heart failure, a murmur of valvular disease a pericardial rub suggesting pericarditis
Measure the patient's blood pressure, both systolic and diastolic values.

Management:
Obtain venous access; take bloods for investigations and blood grouping and cross-matching.
Give a rapid fluid challenge (over 5–10 minutes), reassess the pulse rate and BP regularly (every 5 minutes), watching for signs of improvement.
If not already done, consider inserting a urinary catheter.
In patients with known cardiac failure, early consideration should be given to invasive monitoring.
If the patient shows no signs of improvement, the fluid challenge can be repeated. Consider other causes of shock, get expert help.

5.3. *(see pages 115–116)*
Ensure patent airway, give high flow oxygen. If unable to clear, get help.
Check adequacy of ventilation, monitor SpO_2.
Assess circulation; pulse, BP, CRT, obtain venous access, check blood sugar, take bloods for routine tests plus toxicology. ECG monitor. Arterial blood gases.
Assess neurological state; eye opens to pain = 2, Inappropriate words = 3, localises to pain = 5, GCS = 10.
The small pupils suggest the possibility of opiate overdose, check for evidence of drug abuse (needle marks). Consider giving naloxone. May need respiratory support.
Needs admitting to level 2 care.

5.4. *(see pages 117–118)*
Assess the patient's responsiveness, (don't forget to put on gloves)
Confirm cardiac arrest: look, listen, feel for breathing for up to 10 s, while checking for a carotid pulse.

Start CPR, 30 compressions followed by 2 ventilations. Get member of staff to call the cardiac arrest team and collect resuscitation equipment and a defibrillator.

Attach monitor/defibrillator or AED as soon as possible.

Defibrillate if appropriate or continue CPR.

Hand over to the cardiac arrest team leader when the team arrives.

5.5. (*see pages 121–122*)

Immediate defibrillation using a single shock of 150–200 J if biphasic, 360 J if monophasic.

Restart CPR without checking for a pulse or reassessing the rhythm and continue for 2 minutes after which pause briefly to check the monitor.

If VF/VT persists give second shock, 150–360 J biphasic, 360 J monophasic.

Immediately restart CPR for 2 minutes after which pause briefly to check the monitor.

If VF/VT persists give 1 mg adrenaline IV followed immediately by third shock, 150–360 J biphasic, 360 J monophasic.

Restart CPR for 2 minutes after which pause briefly to check the monitor.

If VF/VT persists, give 300 mg amiodarone IV, followed immediately by third shock, 150–360 J biphasic, 360 J monophasic.

6. Management of the critically ill patient

6.1. (*see page 113*)

Blood pressure is usually measured invasively by the percutaneous insertion of a cannula into an artery. The arterial blood pressure is transmitted to a pressure transducer that converts the mechanical signal to a very small electrical signal, proportional to the pressure. This signal is amplified and displayed on a monitor as both a waveform and as pressure readings: systolic, diastolic and mean.

Advantages:

Accuracy, particularly at high and low pressure.

Continuous.

Shape of arterial waveform gives information relating to myocardial contractility Allows frequent arterial blood sampling.

Disadvantages:

Requires expertise for insertion and care.

Inaccurate if not calibrated.

Haematoma and infection at puncture site.

Disconnection haemorrhage.

Damage to artery.

6.2. (*see page 113*)

Indications for inserting a central venous catheter:

Measurement of central venous pressure.

To infuse irritant solutions, vasoconstrictor drugs, give parenteral nutrition.

To allow insertion of temporary cardiac pacing wire.

To allow venous access for haemodialysis, haemofiltration, plasmaphoresis etc.

Lack of suitable peripheral veins.

Complications:

Puncture of adjacent artery or damage to other local structures (poor technique).

Haematoma, infection/septicaemia.

Pneumothorax (most likely with subclavian approach) hence always get a CXR postprocedure.

Air embolism.

6.3. (*see pages 144–145*)

Risk factors for nosocomial infection:

The elderly and very young.

Pre-existing medical conditions.

Poor nutritional status.

Patients who are immunosuppressed.

Where there are breeches of body surface defences; intubation, urinary catheterisation, IV lines.

Use of H2-antagonists or PPIs to prevent gastric ulceration.

Prevention:

Good basic hygiene standards; hand washing, wearing of gloves and aprons.

Regular disinfection of ventilator tubing or use of disposable equipment.

Insertion of IV lines, catheters with full aseptic technique.

Ensuring that surgical wounds and sites of insertion of IV lines, catheters are kept clean.

Bacterial/viral filters between patient and ventilator.

Avoid overuse of 'prophylactic' broad-spectrum antibiotics.

Optimize nutritional status of patient.

6.4. (*see pages 150–151*)

SIRS is diagnosed on finding two or more of the following:

- Temperature >38°C or <36°C.
- Heart rate >90 beats/min.
- Tachypnoea >20 breaths/min or $PaCO_2$ <32 mmHg.
- White blood cell count $>12 \times 10^9$/L, or $<4 \times 10^9$/L, or >10% immature forms.

Key interventions in the first 6 hours:

IV access, routine bloods, blood cultures, arterial blood gases, lactate.

Fluid bolus, 20 ml/kg if mean arterial pressure <65 mmHg or serum lactate concentration >4 mmol/l with further boluses according to response.

Start a vasopressor (eg noradrenaline) via a central line if no response to fluid challenges.

Achieve and maintain central venous pressure >11 cm H_2O.

Administer antibiotics within three hours of presentation.

Achieve and maintain central venous oxygen saturation ($S_{CV}O_2$) > 70%.

6.5. (*see pages 138–139*)

Indications for mechanical ventilation on ICU:

Established respiratory failure or impending failure in an exhausted patient.

Patients who are hypoxic ($PaO_2 \leq 8$ kPa) with or without accompanying hypercapnia ($PaCO_2 \geq$ 6.6 kPa).

Patients with ARDS.

Head injured patients where ventilation may be part of the regimen to control intracranial pressure

Gas exchange improved by:

Allows 100% oxygen to be given.

Reduces oxygen consumption.

Ventilation with larger tidal volumes, variable rates.

Allows the use of PEEP to increase the FRC.

In the failing heart, reduces both preload and afterload, improving cardiac output.

May reduce pulmonary oedema.

6.6. (*see pages 140–141*)

Patients with an acute exacerbation of chronic obstructive pulmonary disease (COPD). The benefits are clearer in more severe exacerbations (pH < 7.3, PCO2 > 6 kPa), patients of younger age, unimpaired level of consciousness and a prompt positive response within the first few hours.

Advantages:

The patient remains conscious, without the need for sedation and a tracheal tube.

ICU admission is not mandatory, can be done in HDU.

The patient breaths spontaneously (with positive pressure assistance).

Weaning is usually easier and more successful.

The risk of ventilator-associated pneumonia (VAP) is reduced.

Speech and eating retained.

Disadvantages:

The mask is tight-fitting and may not tolerated.

No airway protection, risk of aspiration.

Need a cooperative patient with reasonable respiratory effort.

Ventilatory support limited.

Risk of gastric distention.

Does not allow bronchial toilet.

Index

Page numbers in *italics* refer to figures and those in **bold** to tables; note that figures and tables are only indicated when they are separated from their text references.

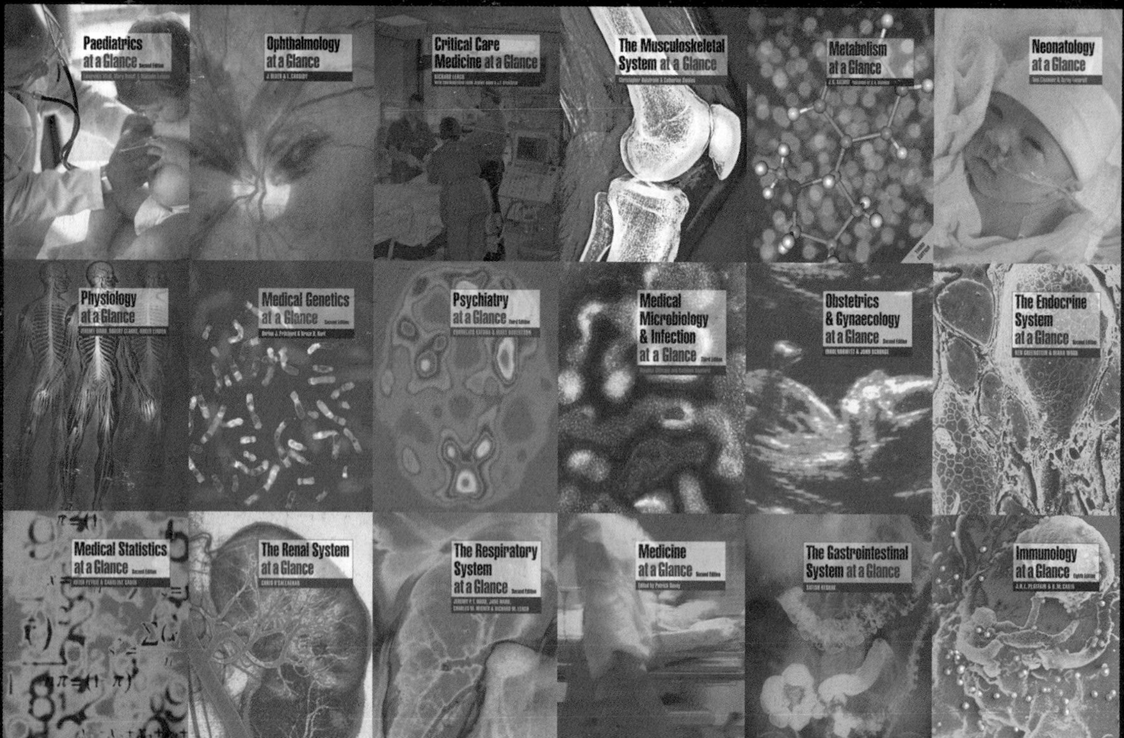